Tribal Health in Eastern Ghats

About the Author

Prof. K.E. Rajpramukh obtained degrees of M.A. and Ph.D. in Anthropology from Andhra University. Having taught at many universities, he was also on the Guest Faculty at the University of Hyderabad. He joined the University of Rochester, NY, U.S.A. as a Research Associate in 1988 and pursued his Master's Degree in Public Health from the School of Medicine and Dentistry at the same University during 1990 and 1993. He was Chairman, Board of Studies in Anthropology of Andhra University during 1999-2002.

He has authored five books including *Medical Anthropology, Health, Illness and Healing and Dalit Christians of Andhra with contribution of publishing several research papers in national and international journals of repute.*

Tribal Health in Eastern Ghats

K.E. Rajpramukh

CONCEPT PUBLISHING COMPANY Pvt. Ltd.
NEW DELHI-110059

ISBN-13 : 978-81-8069-841-5

First Published 2012

Published and Printed by

Concept
Since 1974

Concept Publishing Company Pvt. Ltd.
A/15-16, Commercial Block, Mohan Garden
New Delhi-110059 (India)
T: 25351460, 25351794, *F*: 091-11-25357109
E: publishing@conceptpub.com, W: www.conceptpub.com
Editorial Office: H-13, Bali Nagar, New Delhi-110 015, India.

Cataloging in Publication Data--*Courtesy:* D.K. Agencies (P) Ltd. <docinfo@dkagencies.com>

Rajpramukh, K. E.
Tribal health in Eastern Ghats / K.E. Rajpramukh.
p. cm.
Includes bibliographical references (p.) and index.
ISBN 9788180698415

1. Eastern Ghats (India)—Scheduled tribes—Medical care. 2. Primary health care—India—Eastern Ghats. I. Title.

DDC 362.109548 23

Preface

Anthropological research in health and illness is a relatively recent trend despite the fact that a substantial body of beliefs, knowledge and practices in every society is built around the major life experiences of health and illness. Ackernecht (1947) has rightly pointed out: "Disease and its treatment are only in the abstract purely biological processes. Actually, such facts whether a person gets sick at all, what kind of disease he acquires and what kind of treatment he receives depend largely upon social factors". The significant links between human behaviour and disease etiology and transmission have been recognized for many years as illustrated in the works of Alland (1972), Dunn (1976 , 1979 and 1983), Hesser (1982) , Polgar (1964) and Roundy (1978).

Ill-health is a universal human experience. But the distribution of diseases in kind and magnitude varies from society to society and this variance could be explained with the help of different biological, ecological and socio-cultural factors. Alland (1972) studied how cultural practices could be used to promote health and hygiene. Drawing upon the concept from mathematical modelling, he used the term 'minimax' to refer to cultural behaviours that minimize the risk of disease and maximize the health of the groups. However, in case of tribals in India it is found that many of their behavioural practices are not in consonance with this model.

It is too well known that the tribals lag behind enormously in many areas including health compared to other populations in India and poverty obviously is at the root of the problem besides other socio-cultural factors. As there is no comprehensive work on the Tribals of Eastern Ghats with respect to their health status an attempt is made here to criticaliy examine the ill-health experiences of the tribals and the functioning of the existing health care facilities available to them.

Acknowledgements

The study of health and illness is a challenging task as it involves many facets of human experience. The health status of the tribals is mired in many a factor including their belief systems related to their conceptions of health and illness. As differences exist between various tribal communities in their socio-cultural practices related to health and illness despite some basic similarities developing a tribal health policy is fraught with careful handling. As this study is undertaken toward that goal substantial financial support to carry out such a task becomes immanent. In this connection I am extremely grateful to the Ministry of Tribal Affairs, Government of India, for funding this Project.

I am also thankful to all the tribals who participated in this study and the Staff of the PHCs covered in this study. My grateful thanks are also due to the ITDA Officers, Tribal Welfare Officers, and the Medical Officers in all the districts covered under the study. Rich secondary data were collected with the cooperation of the Department of Anthropology at Utkal University and the Tribal Research Institute at Bhubaneswar. My grateful thanks to all those associated with these institutions.

This study would not have been accomplished without the active participation of our Research scholars, viz., Suribabu, Appala Naidu, Laxminarayana, Sanyasi Naidu and Jhansi Rani. I happily acknowledge their contribution to this study in the collection of data, tabulation and compilation.

Visakhapatnam **Prof. K.E. Rajpramukh**
9th April 2010

EASTERN GHATS

Rivers	Godavari • Kaveri • Krishna • Mahanadi • Palar • Ponnaiyar • Sweata Nadi • Vasishta Nadi • Vellar
Regions	Deccan Plateau • Kolar Plateau
Hills	Bilgiri (Biligirirangan) • Chitteri • Kalrayan • Karanthamalai • Kolli • Lankamalla • Mettur • Nallamalla • Pachaimalai • Palamalai • Palikonda • Shevaroy • Sirumalai • Vada Chennimalai • Velikonda
Waterfalls	Kiliyur • Periyar • Pudur Megan • Mayil Uthu • Mangalam • Agaya Gangai
States	Andhra Pradesh • Orissa • Tamil Nadu • West Bengal

Contents

List of Tables

I
Introduction

WHO defines Health as: 'Health is a state of complete physical, mental and social well-being and not merely the absence of disease or infirmity'.

India has the second largest tribal population in the world, next to Africa. There are 630 tribes, sub-divided into groups, spread over the length and breadth of the country, concentrated mostly in the hilly and forest regions. The tribal population of India, as per the 2001 census, is 8.43 crore, constituting 8.2 per cent of the total population. The population of tribes had grown at the rate of 24.45 per cent during the period 1991-2001. More than half the Scheduled Tribe population is concentrated in the States of Madhya Pradesh, Chattisgarh, Maharashtra, Orissa, Jharkhand and Gujarat. Tribal communities live in about 15 per cent of the country's areas, in various ecological and geo-climatic conditions ranging from plains and forests to hills and inaccessible areas. Tribal groups are at different stages of social, economic and educational development. Some tribal communities have been thoroughly acculturated and adopted a mainstream way of life. At the other end of the spectrum, there are certain scheduled tribes known as Primitive Tribal Groups (PTGs), who are characterized by, a pre-agriculture level of technology; a stagnant or declining population; extremely low literacy; and a subsistence level of economy (Tribal Affairs, 2006-2007).

Tribe

In English the word 'tribe' came to be used for those tribes of Israel since the middle of the thirteenth century. The Oxford English dictionary (1989) defines it as "a group of persons forming a community and claiming descent from a common ancestor". By the beginning of the fifteenth century usage of the term extended to include "lineage" or 'line of descent' and was, therefore, regularly applied to descriptions of Irish social groups who were 'families or communities' of persons having the same surname.

The term 'primitive tribe' was often used by western anthropologists to denote "A primary aggregate of peoples living in a primitive or barbarous condition under a headman or chief." (Lewis, 1972: 146). Some Anthropologists defined tribe as a people at earlier stage of evolution of society. This gave a sort of moral tone that the tribals are yet to develop and become civilized. It is because of this that they were also known as 'primitive' 'barbarous' or aboriginal people. This sort of moralistic overtone was later on reduced with the usage of terms like 'pre-state society', 'pre-literate society' or 'simple society'. All these terms with evolutionary idiom indicated that the tribes are backward in comparison to other populations. In this sense tribal development means a transformation from pre-state to state society, from pre-literate to literate society, from simple to complex society and the like.

In the census report of 1891, they were classified under 'forest tribes' (numbering about 16 million) within 'Agricultural and pastoral castes'. In 1901, they were reported as 'Animists' and in 1911 tribal animists or people following tribal religion. According to Singh (1997: 35) "the definition of tribe first appeared in Risley and Gaits 'Census of India, 1901'. A tribe as we find it in India is a collection of families or groups of families, bearing a common name which as a rule does not denote any specific occupation, generally claiming common descent from a mythical or historical ancestor and occasionally from an animal, but in some parts of the country, held together rather by the obligations of blood-fend than by the tradition of kinship, usually speaking the same language and occupying professing or claiming to occupy a definite tract of country. "A tribe is not necessarily endogamous, that is to say, it is not an invariable rule that a man of a particular tribe must marry a woman of that tribe and cannot marry a woman of different tribe".

In 1921, they became "Hill and Forest Tribes" and in 1931 'Primitive Tribes'. The Government of India Act of 1935 classed them as 'Backward Tribes'. The Census of 1941 classed them as 'tribes'; under the Constitution of India certain tribes have been specified as the scheduled tribes.

Only those tribes, which have been included in the list of scheduled tribes, are given special treatment or facilities under the Constitution. Certain tribes, for instance, nomadic tribes, are not specified as scheduled tribes. The Constitution neither defines nor lays down any criteria for specifying the scheduled tribes. As per Article 366 (255) of the Constitution, the scheduled tribes mean such tribes or tribal communities or parts of or groups within such tribes or tribal communities as are deemed under Article 342 to be scheduled tribes for the purposes of this Constitution. The President of India from time to time under Article 342 through a public notification specifies the scheduled tribes. The Parliament may, by law, include or exclude from the list of scheduled tribes any tribal community or part thereof in any State or Union Territory" (Verma, 1990: 10). Verma sums up that the scheduled tribes must have the following features :

1. The traditional occupation and a geographical area.
2. A distinctive culture including language, customs, traditions, religious beliefs, arts, crafts, etc.
3. A primitive occupation, economy, etc.
4. Lack of education and techno-economic development.

Grigson argued effectively in favour of special measures for aboriginals. According to him, the primitive tribes were the most backward and the worst exploited communities in India and also the least adapted to the impact of modern conditions. They have their own distinct culture, language, social organization and traditions. "It is remarkable that in his day he advocated co-operatives where tribes men would handle all branches of trade in forest produce, purchase and distribution of consumer goods needed by them as well as panchayats which would ensure a real upward stream of power, from primary voters, through panchayat members to local bodies and legislature" (Grigson, 1946: 81-96).

The concept of Tribe varies from State to State or area to area depending upon local socio-economic conditions of particular community and the consequent inclusion of a particular group in the list of Scheduled Tribes or Scheduled Castes in one State and the same may be backward class or forward class in another State.

For example, *Lambadas* (also known as, *Banjaras* or *Sugalis*) are Scheduled Tribes in Andhra Pradesh, but they are classified as Scheduled Castes in Karnataka and the Union Territory of Delhi and Backward Class in neighbouring Maharashtra. *Korcha* community, which is synonymous of *Yerukula* tribe, is in the list of Scheduled Castes in Karnataka State whereas in Andhra Pradesh, they are listed as Scheduled Tribe. Similarly, *'Goundu'* is a Scheduled Tribe within the Agency tracts of Andhra Pradesh but they are not recognized as a Scheduled Tribe in the adjoining State of Orissa even though they are predominantly found in tribal areas. These kinds of anomalies sometimes encourage migration of identical community from a State where they are not Scheduled tribe/caste, to a State where the same group is Scheduled Tribe/ Caste, in order to draw the benefits accorded to Scheduled Tribes by the Constitution of India.

The Tribal Scenario in India

The tribes differ considerably from one another in race, language, culture, customs and traditions, in their myths and beliefs, and present a spectacle of striking diversity. This diversity, marked by varied racial characteristics and diverse cultural traditions and linguistic traits lend lustre to the cultural mosaic of our country and they represent the true synthesis of India's culture. Each of the tribal groups is a proud community participating in the national life yet retaining its own identity.

In spite of much diversity, there are certain broad similarities between the mutually divergent groups. Striking similarities are noticed in their way of habitation, mode of living, social customs of marriage and divorce, religious beliefs, performance of festivals. It ordinarily has a leader, an ancestor as well as village deity. A tribal society is usually small, isolated, closely knit and is largely organized on the basis of kinship. The most important common feature is their simplicity, honesty and truthfulness.

As an ethnic category having corporate self-identity, Tribes still have a wide range of commonly shared traits of culture like common descent, a collective self-image, possessing distinctive cultural ethos shared by them collectively which gives them a measure of cohesion and unity. Man-nature relationship, magic and sorcery, animist religion, earth, sun, moon, stars and natural phenomenon, ancestral gods, observance of combined feasting, are some of the many common features among all tribals. In spite of the fact that some tribals have adopted Christianity their customary traditional institutions are still intact.

Looking at the diverse cultural traditions and beliefs of the tribals, after attainment of independence, much thought has gone into developing them to a level with the rest of the people—socially, economically, culturally and politically. Before independence, landlords, zamindars, forest contractors, liquor vendors, revenue excise and police officials, moneylenders, and merchants exploited tribals. The British rulers who followed the policy of *laissez-faire* in respect of the tribals left them in isolation. The British policy transformed the tribal's relationship with the forest. Tribals had depended on forests for food, fuel and cattle feed. They practiced shifting cultivation, known as *podu.* The Government usurped forest lands and placed restrictions. Oppression and extortion by policemen, petty officials and moneylenders further aggravated distress among the tribals.

After independence, it was the problem of integration and consolidation. There can be two ways of approaching the problem of tribal people. One is called the 'Anthropological approach' of treating these people as museum specimen, to be observed and written about, and not as living human beings with whom one could work and play. The other approach is of rather ignoring that they are something special and different and trying to absorb them into the normal pattern of society. Both these approaches are wrong. Neither the 'museum approach' nor 'open-door approach' can succeed but we have to find a middle course. We must give them a measure of protection in their areas so that no outsider can interfere with them except with their consent and goodwill. They have to progress in their own way. They do not like something alien to be imposed upon them. No individual can grow in alien surroundings, habits or customs. We have to make them progress but progress does not mean an attempt merely to duplicate what we have got in other parts of India. What is good for the rest of India, will of course, be adopted by them gradually. Imposition should be absent and people have to be trained to train others. Progress may not be rapid. It will definitely take its time.

The Eastern Ghats

Eastern Ghats in South India are a rugged, long chain of broken hills and mountain ranges running almost parallel to the eastern coast of India, and constitutes the watershed of many big rivers. The Eastern Ghats are broadly spread over three States, i.e., Southern Orissa Highlands, coastal Andhra Pradesh and Nilgiri region of Tamil Nadu.

The southern Orissa highlands comprise the Dandakaranya region of Orissa, which includes the districts of Bolangir, Ganjam, Phulbani, Kalahandi, Koraput and part of Puri. The average rainfall in this region is between 2,000-3,000 mm. As per the 2001 census of the total tribal population of India is 84.33 million of which 10.84 per cent live in Orissa. A total of 62 tribal groups constitute 22.1 per cent of the State's total population. The most populous tribes are Gond, Santhal, Oraon, and Kondh and some of the typical tribes like Bhuiyan, Bondo and Juang are found only in Orissa. Mayurbhanj district has the highest concentration of tribals with 57.87 per cent and Khurda district has the lowest with 0.23 per cent (1991 census). Of the 33 scheduled tribes in Andhra Pradesh, 22 live in Eastern Ghats. Some of the prominent tribes of Eastern Ghats are, the *Bagata, Gadaba, Jatapu, Savara, Konda Dora, Khond, Valmiki, Koya, Chenchus, Konda Reddys,* etc. The hill ranges of Cuddapah district in the Rayalaseema region form the central portion of the Eastern Ghats, and the district is drained mainly by the Pennar river and its tributaries. The average annual rainfall here is 685 mm. The Eastern Ghats in Tamil Nadu cover Dharmapuri, North Arcot, Salem and Nilgiri districts. The uplands and the Nilgiri region of Tamil Nadu have wide valleys made by the river Cauvery and its tributaries. In general, the elevation here is over 900 metres in the west due to the Nilgiri hills. The western and eastern flanks get an annual rainfall of 800-2,000 mm but the central part of the uplands is almost dry.

Tribal Health

Generally speaking, the health status of the Tribals is very low compared to other population groups. Poverty undoubtedly is the root cause of morbidity and mortality. Infant mortality rates vary from 120 to 150 per 1000 population whereas it is 72 per 1000 in the general population. Maternal mortality is 8 per 1000, going up to 25 in some primitive tribal groups, as against 4 per 1000 for the State of Andhra Pradesh (Sujatha Rao, 1998). The crude death rate is 15-20 per 1000 with children under 5 accounting for more than 50 per cent of the deaths, whereas it is 9 per 1000 for the general population with children under 5 accounting for 30 per cent of the deaths. Longevity is lower and the incidence rate of TB is double among the Tribals compared to the general population. In a survey (Rajpramukh, 2001) conducted on the Tribals of Vizianagaram district in 2001, it was found that infant mortality rate was between 12-15 per 1000 whereas the current national figure was 4 per 1000. In some of the primitive tribes like the *Savaras* and *Porjas* it was found to be more than 25 per 1000. These findings suggest inter-tribal differentials with regard to their health status. There could also be gender-based differentials in this regard as there is paucity of literature in this area.

The traditional tribal medicine man (the shaman) plays an important role in curing the tribal diseases. He tends to locate the cure and cause of the disease in the same supernatural source (Rajpramukh, 2005). For him the wrath of the supernatural anger causes the disease and the appeasement of the same supernatural power through sacrifice and prayer restores the health of the victim. It is believed that the locally available herbal/ethno-medicine possessed healing power because of the prayers recited and rituals performed by the shaman. Invoking divine beings for blessings is a common practice among many populations including the tribals at the time of agricultural operations. In the area of health and disease too, dependence on divinatory forces is distinctly visible in the tribals' curative practices. The shamanistic practice is age old and the tribal for centuries was left with no other alternative. The role and functions of the Tribal Medicine man is dealt with elaborately in Chapter IV.

Over a period of time, our conceptualization of Health Care also has witnessed shifts as we started with 'Basic Health Services' in 1946 and moved to 'Primary Health Care' in 1979 (Qadeer, 1995). As per the Constitution, the State has to provide basic health care to all its citizens and provisioning of health care services was perceived to be a function of establishing health care institutions according to a population norm. "Accordingly, for every 3,000 population a sub-centre (SC) was established and for every 20,000 population a primary health centre (PHC) as opposed to the norm of 5,000 and 30,000 respectively for non-tribal areas. Accordingly, as on today, there are in the tribal areas, 111 PHCs and 823 SCs along with 29 mobile medical units (MMU), 21 hospitals and 18 dispensaries" (Sujata Rao : 482)

One good thing that followed the 1978 Alma Ata declaration was the proliferation of Primary Health Centres (PHCs) in tribal areas making *allopathy* medicines widely available. In Andhra Pradesh, in places like Paderu, Ayurveda and Homoeopathy hospitals also were established. There is also the presence of private Ayurveda and Homoeo practitioners in certain tribal areas. The Government of Andhra Pradesh has recently announced that in every PHC all these alternative medicines also would be made available in future. In many tribal areas in India at present medicine is being administered by different specialists practicing different medical systems in addition to the native medicine man. Therefore, the tribals once left with no other alternative except to receive treatment from the traditional medicine man are now provided with a number of alternatives in seeking medical treatment.

Some Physical and Genetic Characteristics of Andhra Pradesh Tribals

Many studies conducted on the Eastern Ghats tribals of north coastal Andhra Pradesh brought to light the physical/genetic characteristics of these tribal populations. According to a study on the anthropometry of tribals of Visakhapatnam agency area (Mythili, 1988) the mean body weight among the Konda Dora females is 39.46 ± 0.38 against the measurements of 36.69 ± 0.15 to 42.79 ± 0.60 among the Andhra female population. The Konda Kammaras come closer to Gadabas. Kondadoras are usually short with the average height of 147.73 ± 0.40 cm against the mean stature of 148.91 ± 0.49 to 150.37 ± 0.44cm in case of Andhra females. The Konda Dora females are found to be closer to the Gadabas and Samanthas. The sitting height among the Konda Dora females is an average of 73.62 ± 0.41 cm against the Andhra average of 72.50 ± 0.29 to 81.04 ± 0.37 cm. In this respect the Konda Dora females are very close to Konda Reddies and Koya Doras.

Regarding the arm length most of the Konda Doras come under 65.1-70.0 cm category with average for females at 68.64 ± 0.27 cm.

The average bio-cranial diameter among females is 32.40 ± 0.13 cm against the 28.69 ± 0.15 to 32.11 cm for Andhra population. In this respect the Konda Dora females are closer to Samanthas.

The mean transverse chest breadth among Konda Dora females is 24.35 ± 0.13 cm, the antero-posterior chest girth is 19.63 ± 0.11 cm, and the mean bi-Iliocrystal diameter is 25.85 ± 0.23 cm. For morphological facial height majority of the females are in very high and high categories. The average value for females is 11.79 ± 0.04 cm against the Andhra measurements of 9.53 ± 0.55 to 10.73 ± 0.05 cm. The Konda Dora females come closer to Jathapus and Konda Kammaras.

Regarding the maximum head breadth most of the Konda Dora females belong to the very narrow category with the average value being 13.00 ± 0.03 cm whereas it varies from 12.07 ± 0.05 to 13.41 ± 0.05 cm for the Andhra Population. In this the Konda Dora females come closer to Konda Reddies and Konda Kammaras. Females usually show long heads and the mean for maximum head length for Konda Dora females is 18.90 ± 0.03 against the Andhra figures for the same as 17.27 cm ± 0.05 to 18.23 ± 0.07 cm. In this regard the Konda Dora females come closer to Lambadas and Porangi Porjas.

Most of the Konda Dora females come under the narrow category for breadth of Bizygomatic arch with the average values of 12.18 ± 0.03 cm against the values for Andhra population being 10.61 ± 0.57 to 12.51 ± 0.05 cms. The Konda Dora females some what resemble Porangi Porja tribe in this regard.

The mean upper arm circumference of Konda Dora females is 29.98 ± 0.14 cm. The mean value for triceps skinfold is 45.59 ± 0.07 cm and the value for mean in subscapular skinfold measurement is 6.38 ± 0.11 cm.

Seven body indices have been calculated using the 15 measurements taken, some of which are compared with the available data on other populations of Andhra Pradesh. The average values for relative sitting height index is 49.88 ± 0.12 cm. For relative sitting height index majority of females come under Macroskel category. The mean values are ranging from 48.13 ± 0.33 cm to 50.11 cm in other tribal populations. Regarding this index value Konda Doras are somewhat closer to Konda Reddies and Samantha Tribes. With regard to relative biacromial breadth index most of the females fall under long arm class. The average value is 21.93 cm ± 0.2 cm. The average values of Andhra populations are ranging from 18.94 ± 0.16 to 21.82 ± 0.21 cm. In this Konda Doras are closer to Samanthas.

The mean values observed for thoracic index is 60.96 ± 0.63 cm. Most of them come under the category of 74.0-84.9 cm type against the Andhra Pradesh figures of 51.49 ± 0.18 cm to 54.56 ± 0.28 cm. In this regard the Konda Doras are closer to Samanthas.

For cephalic index majority of the Konda Dora females are hyper dolicocephalic and dolicocephalic. The mean value is 72.25 ± 0.28 cm against the Andhra Pradesh figures of 72.15 ± 0.32-84.01 ± 0.19 cm. They are closer to Konda Reddies and Samanthas.

The most frequent category of morphological facial index is hyperleptoprosophic. The mean value is 95.74 ± 0.70 cm against the Andhra Pradesh figure of 83.30-106.71 cm in females. Majority of females fall in 'long arm class' for relative upper extremity index and the mean value is 43.93 ± 0.12 cm. The mean value of Pandoral index is 24.14 ± 1.04 cm against the Andhra Pradesh figures of 23.11 ± 0.06 to 23.58 ± 0.06 cm.

A study (Laxmi, 1977) of genetic demography on the Konda Kammara tribe of Addatheegala block in East Godavari district in Andhra Pradesh demonstrates the following findings on the basis of 150 women. The age at marriage of the Konda Kammara females is 12-14 years with a preference for consanguineous marriages. The age at first conception is between 15 and 19 years and the last between 25-29 years. The infant mortality rate is found to be very high at 58.46 per cent. The age at menopause is 45 years. Among them fertility appears to rise with the increasing duration of marriage. The women who marry late tend to account for their relatively low fertility. This clearly shows the association between high fertility and earlier age at marriage. At the same time the fertility performance of women does not have any significant association with the age at marriage and regional pattern of marriage whereas it is significantly associated with present age of women, duration of married life, pregnancy wastage, mortality of children, family size and family form. The incidence of high fertility is related to older in age, earlier marriage, longer duration of married life, absence of any pregnancy wastage, high mortality, simple form of family. The women generally are weak and anaemic due to malnutrition. Most of the women chew tobacco and even smoke. Personal and household cleanliness is very poor. Diarrhoea is the common disease prevalent among the children. A disease they locally call, *anasa* apparently is the root cause for infant mortality. All diseases among them could be easily attributable to their abject poverty.

Dermatoglyphics

Findings related to Finger and Palm prints of 85 unrelated individuals of Savara males of Bhadragiri agency in Srikakulam district of Andhra Pradesh have been studied (Venkateswarlu, 1975): (1) Finger patterns; whorls: 43.29 per cent; Loop Radial: 1.41 per cent; Loop Ulnar; 52 per cent; Arches: 3.05 per cent; (2) Comparative occurrence of loops and whorls on both hands: Ist digit: L > W; IInd digit: W > L; IIIrd digit: L > W; IVth digit: W > L; and Vth digit: L > W; (3) Pattern intensity index: 2 × W + 1 × L/10 = 13.99 per cent; (4) Arch/Whorl index or Dankneijer's index = Arches/whorls x 100= 7.06 per cent; (5) Whorl/Loop index or Furuhata's index = Whorls/ Loops × 100 = 81.05; (6) Bimanaur: highest peak at whorls 4 and 0 arches= 12.94; (7) Symmetry: 74.35 per cent; (8) Asymmetry: 25.65 per cent; (9) Monomorphic hands—Whorls: 20 per cent; Loop: 30.5 per cent; (10) Pair Group Rule-Validity: Σ P > G: 1.493 (P) –2.99 (G), therefore P > G; (11) Ridge Count: Highest ridge count is 65 occurs in the IVth digit of the right hand; (12) Total ridge count: The highest total ridge count ranges from 441-460 with 1.17 per cent. The highest peak of total ridge count ranges from 141-160 with 11.11 per cent; (13) Range of ridge count in ten digits—right hand: IV > III > I > V > II; Left Hand: III > IV > I > II > V; (14) Mean: 19.98 per cent; (15) Standard deviation: 185.83 per cent; (16) Standard error of mean= 6.37 per cent; (17) Coefficient of variation: 930.08 per cent; (18) S.E. of S.D= 4.5 per cent; (19) S.E. of C.V.=22.56 per cent.

Palmar Dermatoglyphics

(20) Main lines: 7, 5″, 5″, 4 with 12.94 per cent; 9, 7, 5 ′ 4 with 12.35 per cent; 11, 9, 7, 4 with 11.17 per cent; (21) Wilder's three main line formulae: 11, 9, 7 with 25.88 per cent; 9, 7, 5, with 21.17 per cent; 7, 5, 5 with 18.82 per cent; 11, 9, 7 > 9, 7, 5 > 7, 5, 5; (22) Three model types of line D—Left: MT-9 > M.T.-7 > M.T.-7; (23) Three model types of line A—Left: MT-3 > M.T.-1 >M.T.-5; Right: M.T.-3 > M.T._5 > M.T.-1; (24) Endings of main lines d, c, b, and A : D ends in 7,8,9,10,11; C ends in 5′5″, 6,7,9,10,11; ends in 4, 5′, 5″, 6,7,8,9; A

ends in 1,2,3,4,5,5". (25) Main line index values—8=24.7 per cent; 6=21.15 per cent; 10=19.4 per cent; 11=14.7 per cent; (26) Axial triradii= t= 77.05 per cent; t'=17.05 per cent; t"= 2.35 per cent; (27) Hypothenar: A=37.05 per cent; V=20.58 per cent; A/A=15.88 per cent; (28) Thenar and Ist interdigits—A=62.93 per cent; O=21.74 per cent; M=13.52 per cent; V=1.76 per cent; (29) Interdigital II= O=87.64 per cent; V=5.53 per cent; D=2.93 per cent; (30) Interdigital III—O=68.23 per cent; L=13.52 per cent; O/1=11.15 per cent; (31) Interdigital IV—O=29.41 per cent; L=22.35 per cent; O/1=7.9 per cent; V=6.46 per cent; O/L=4.79 per cent.

In a study on three genetic disorders, viz., Sickle cell trait, Glucose-6-phosphate dehydrogenase (G6PD) deficiency. among the tribals of Andhra Pradesh, Veerraju (1984: 143) points out that high incidence of sickle cell gene in the hetero zygous condition is found among the tribals than the caste population on account of malarial endemicity in the tribal areas which is responsible for the natural selection of this trait. Highest incidence of G6PD deficiency is reported among the Koya Doras. Colour blindness was reported high among the Valmikis followed by Konda Reddy, Koya Dora, Bagatha in that order

In a study on the morbidities among the tribals of Vizianagaram Sub-Plan area, Andhra Pradesh, (1998) it was found that among all the illnesses reported fevers occupy the top position followed by scabies and respiratory diseases. Stagnant pools of water prove to be the breeding places for mosquitoes which cause malaria. Skin infections, mostly scabies, seem to be high among the children in the age group of 5-15 due to insufficient washing of hands and feet after play and the incidence is high in the months of February, March, April and May in which there usually is acute shortage of water. Body pains are due to carrying head loads of their daily necessities of water and firewood. Worm infestations are due to consumption of contaminated water.

In a study (2006: 32-47) on child health care among the Santals of the Midnapore District of West Bengal, Pinak Tarafdar pointed out three factors such as 'place of delivery, polio vaccination and availing of ICDS facilities' as crucial to child health care.

Nutrition among the Tribals

According to Kreuter (1980), Nutrition is both a process and a science. Thus, nutrition as the biological process, deals with the mechanisms by which humans utilize food to meet the requirements of biological and behavioural functioning. Moreover as a science it studies the whole gamut of the body's chemical processing and biological use of food. The Council of Food and Nutrition defines nutrition (1963) as, "the science of food, the nutrients and other substances therein, their action, interaction and balance in relation to health and disease and the process by which the organism ingests, absorbs, transports, utilizes and executes food substances. In addition, nutrition must be concerned with social, economic, cultural and psychological implication of food and eating".

Nutritional status can be measured in two ways: one, based on 'input' indicators such as food and nutrient intake, and the other, based on 'output' indicators such as anthropometry (e.g., height, weight and arm circumference) and clinical signs (e.g., colour of eyes and hair, and Hb level) showing ill effects of nutritional intake. Between the input and output indicators, the input indicators can vary quickly while the output indicators are relatively more stable over a period except in case of sudden, severe illness. Further, the data needed to measure the output indicators can be obtained from single survey whereas a variety of methods are needed to measure the input indicators. 'Gomez' classification of different grade of malnutrition is being substituted in India by a classification system as recommended by Indian Academy of Paediatricians (IAP, 1972) keeping in view the growth pattern in Indian children.

It is shocking to note that 63.3 per cent of Bonda children during harvesting season and 75 per cent of the Bonda children during lean season are malnourished. The incidence of Grade III and Grade IV malnutrition among Bonda children is 10.5 per cent in lean season and the same is 6.3 per cent in harvesting season. Except intake of nutrients such as calcium, iron, Vitamin A, Vitamin B1, Vitamin B2, the consumption of other essential nutrients namely calorie, protein and Vitamin C among the Bonda is not at all satisfactory and falls short of recommended allowances.

Child death rate is the number of deaths of children aged 1-4 years per 1,000 children in the same age group in a given year. It thus excludes infant mortality. Jhansi Rani (2009) reports that the child death rate among the Bondos is 207 against the State figure of 148.8 for tribal population and 175.8 for the scheduled caste population. Inter-village variation of child death rate among the studied population is very prominent. The highest child death rate is observed at Badbel (390) followed by Bandhuguda (320) in Malkangiri district.

The major causes of high child death rate are lack of immunization, diarrhoea, ARI, malaria and moreover high incidence of severe malnutrition accelerates the vulnerability of child population in Bondo society.

Tribal Communities of Orissa

Orissa, one of the States in Eastern India, is famous for harbouring 62 tribal communities and it occupies the second place in India in terms of concentration of tribal population (Nearly 23%).

The composition of diet of most of the tribes is extremely simple but a mixed one. It usually consists of boiled rice, millets, or simply gruel made up of the foodgrains with very little quantity of boiled vegetable, pulses and little salt. The consumption of millet is hardly noticed among the Juang of Dhenkanal as they eke out their subsistence partially on wage labour. The Bonda Highlanders consume on an average 4 gm of pulses per day, which is the lowest. The average intake of calorie and protein, the basic nutrients, is quite insufficient, particularly among the Saora (1685 kcl energy; 23.2 gm protein), the Koya (1396 kcl energy; protein 43.6 gm); the Juang (1372.6 kcl energy, protein 32.9 gm); the bonda (1709 kcl, protein 40.2 gm) as against recommended dietary allowance (2400 kcl energy and protein 55 gm) prescribed. However, per day, per unit intake of nutrients of studied tribal groups is not necessarily a true reflection of state of nutrition of the entire population as inter-individual variations across social and economic categories and between seasons are well discernible. One is amazed to observe that the Saora, the Bonda, the Juang and the Koya having been nutritionally under-fed carry out their activities in all kinds of circumstances stringing their body physiology. The trend undoubtedly pose questions about the fundamental premise of balanced nutrition that what should be considered as optimum calorie or protein requirement norm of an individual, by which a man may be called semi-starved or fully starved. There is no denying of the fact that the inadequate consumption of nutrients along side improper assimilation of nutrients due to infection very often lead to reduction in physical growth and development (Mohanty and Das, 2007).

According to a study (Bulliyya, 2006) on Paudi Bhuiyans, who are a neglected group, they are found to be highly disease prone because of hostile environment and poor health care facilities. Their misery is compounded by poverty, illiteracy, ignorance of causes of disease, very poor sanitation, lack of health education and safe drinking water, and faith in traditional beliefs.

The study reports widespread nutritional deficiencies especially the micro-nutrients. Iron deficiency anaemia is widely prevalent in Paudi Bhuiyans with low concentrations of blood hemoglobin (Hb). The proportion of females suffering with different grades of anaemia is more than that of males.

A study by Hemantabag and Kapoor (2007) on the Kondhs of Orissa reports the following diseases during the last six months of their study in this order: Malaria/fever (31.33%); Cough (21.15%); Dysentery (9.14%); Headache (8.09%); Small Pox (5.22%); Typhoid (4.43%); Dental Pain (3.92%); Sore Eyes (3.66%); Scabies (3.39%); and other minor ailments. They seek both traditional and modern means of treatment. Home remedies: Females play an important role. Karanj leaf and custard oil are applied for boils; Saliva is applied for ear pain. If a patient does not get cured within a day or two he/she may be taken to the Baid, Herbalist, gunia or guru (witch doctor), pujari/medical doctor. The role of medicine man and the herbal medicine among the tribals of Eastern Ghats is separately dealt with in Chapters IV and VI respectively.

Studies from Tamil Nadu

In a study on the health status of tribal women and children among eleven tribes of South India, Naidu, *et al.* (2007, 10-27) point out that the age at marriage among the tribal women generally varies from <13 to < 20. Majority of the Malayali Tribe of Yelagiri had their first conception at the age of 16-17 years. Among the Irula it is 18-20 years; while it is 18-19 among the Kurumba and 16-17 years among the Muduga. The same study points out that among the Valmiki of Andhra Pradesh it varies from 16 to 20; and among the Konda Dora it is 16-17 years. The waiting time of these tribal women for their first conception after marriage is 1-2 years for majority of the tribes. Conception immediately after marriage does not pose any problem to health. But conception at a very early age certainly is a problem when many cases of marriage fall between 16-17 years of age. The breast feeding practices among the tribal women indicate removal of colustrum by the tribal women because of their ignorance about it as a good source of nutrients that provides immunity to the child all through its life. The average duration of breast feeding among the Malayali tribe varies from birth up to 6 years. Tubectomy exclusively by all women was reported among them without any vasectomy case.

In a study on health problems related to tobacco culture among the Puniya tribe, Sasicoumar *et al.* (2007) found out that "in Paniya tribe villages, tobacco smoking is done openly among other members of the family including children"(p. 143).

"The health practices among the Paniya are still primitive, based upon legendary beliefs, sickness and poor health are thought to be induced by spirits and gods. Herbs are used to treat the sick, in addition to sacrifices to spirits. Tobacco is known to be effective as medicine for many conditions (p. 144). Since the primary reason for tobacco use is frequently illness and poor health and since tobacco can only suppress the symptoms without curing them, the underlying disease may be masked and continue to progress." (p. 147)

In a study on the food habits and nutritional status on eleven tribes in four southern States in India Dash and Naidu (2007: 150-170) assert that the tribal people irrespective of their places, culture, language and different ecological setting were nutritionally very poor, especially in their calcium, carotene, and iron intake. These are the essential nutrients, calcium for the bone and teeth, leading to deformities in the body structure, teeth, and softness of bone; carotene for the eyes, its deficiency leading to night blindness, a serious hazard to health and other diseases; iron for the formation of blood deficiency, which leads anaemia causing weakness, thereby reducing the working capacity, indirectly affecting the nutritional status of the whole family. So the prevalence of the deficiency of these nutrients has made the incidence of the diseases pertaining to it more and making the tribals a weaker and non-productive contributor to the nation. Nutrition intervention programme, which should be intense has to be implemented to bring the tribals to the main stream of life. (pp. 161-162)

In this background it is proposed to undertake to study the

health status of the tribals inhabiting the Eastern Ghats with the following objectives:

Objectives

1. To construct a profile of tribal diseases and the etiologies;
2. To study the mortality and morbidity rates among the tribals focusing on inter-tribal and gender-based differences;
3. To examine the Health Care Delivery Systems present in the tribal areas including the functioning of P.H.Cs, medical and para-medical staff; and
4. To guide a Public Policy Formulation for Tribal Health.

Methodology

Primary data was collected from the Eastern Ghats Tribals of Andhra Pradesh supplemented by the secondary data collected from Eastern Ghats Tribals inhabiting Orissa and Tamilnadu States. Carefully prepared Schedules for the study of the PHCs located in Tribal areas and also Tribal Villages especially in Andhra Pradesh Eastern Ghats were employed to collect data on all aspects of Primary Health Care. Informal interviews were conducted with the Medical Doctors and Paramedical staff working in tribal areas, including the local medicine-men. All through the study Participant Observation method was the guiding element. Informal interviews and observation were made use in of collecting data pertaining to inter-tribal differences and gender based discrimination, if any. To augment the data thus collected a few case studies on illness episodes and curative practices of tribal patients were recorded. Secondary data generated by the Department of Anthropology, Andhra University, Visakhapatnam, over a period of time also was made use of to supplement the first hand data collected by the field work.

Chapterization

This study was presented in seven chapters. The first Introductory Chapter deals with the statement of the problem drawing insights from the works already done. A brief review of literature is presented here delineating the objectives of this study and the methodology used to collect data.

The second chapter contains the primary data collected from the Eastern Ghats tribal respondents from different villages in different districts of Andhra Pradesh. All aspects related to Primary Health Care are dealt with in this chapter.

The third chapter is on the first hand data collected from the medical staff of the PHCs in the Eastern Ghats of Andhra Pradesh. Aspects related to the administration of Primary Health Care by the Medical Doctors and the supporting staff are dealt with in this chapter.

The fourth chapter deals with the local medicine men in the tribal areas of the Eastern Ghats and their curative practices and the fifth chapter is all about the common diseases that afflict the tribals in the Eastern Ghats.

The sixth chapter deals with the tribal ethno-medicine and the diseases that are cured by their herbal medicine and the last chapter summarises the major findings of this study together with certain recommendations to be taken care of while formulating policies related to tribal health care.

II

Primary Health Care of the Tribals

A carefully prepared village schedule covering different aspects of primary health care and other health details was administered to the villages in the five districts of Eastern Ghats in Andhra Pradesh. Table 2.1 gives information related to the villages studied such as the tribe/tribes inhabiting the village, the total number of households in the village, and the population characteristics.

It can be seen from Table 2.1 that almost all the tribes inhabiting the Eastern Ghats of Andhra Pradesh, viz., Jatapu, Savara, Gadaba, Konda Reddy, Porja, Bagata, Khond, Konda Dora, Valmiki, Konda Kammara, Koya and Sugali were covered. Most of the villages studied were on the hill top which typically contains the Eastern Ghats tribals in Andhra Pradesh. The size of the tribal villages studied varies within a range of 16 to 56, the smallest being Melikavalasa in Vizianagaram District inhabited by the Jatapu tribe and the largest being Vanjara in West Godavari district inhabited by the Konda Reddy and Sugali tribes. The population size falls within a range of 55 and 280 corresponding to the household range. It can be seen from the Table that the females out number males in the population composition in half of the villages especially in case of Jatapus and Koya.

Table 2.2 relates to the educational and economic status, including their occupations and landholdings, of the tribals of the villages studied. It can be seen from Table 2.2 that there are more number of illiterates among them than the literates with the exception of Modapali in Visakhapatnam District which is inhabited by Bagatas; Vanjara in West Godavari District which is

Table 2.1: Demographic Details of the Villages Studied

District	*Village*	*HH*	*TP*	*M*	*F*	*M*	*UM*	*Tribe*			
								Jatapu	*Savara*	*Gadaba*	*Konda Reddy*
Srikakulam	Ulipiri Valasa	48	213	86	127	110	103	48	—	—	—
	Ranga Puram	26	110	44	68	63	46	12	14	—	—
Vizianagaram	Gandinagar	19	80	37	43	55	30	14	—	—	5
	Melikavalasa	16	55	29	26	33	22	16	—	—	—
	Dippavalasa	28	135	66	69	75	58	—	—	28	—
Visakhapatnam	Solabam	24	96	49	47	55	41	Porja	—	—	—
	Modapali	39	156	84	72	95	61	Bagata	—		—
	Injari	28	115	66	49	75	40	Gadaba	—		—
	Doduput	34	162	86	76	98	64	Kondu 14, Konda Dora 20	—	—	—
	Downuru	18	92	45	47	57	35	Valmiki	—	—	—
East Godavari	I. Polavar	42	210	115	95	140	70	Konda Kammara 18	—	—	24
	Kindra	47	235	126	109	186	49	Konda Dora 27 Valmiki 20	—	—	
West Godavari	Kommu. G	22	88	40	48	58	30	Koya	—	—	—
	Vanjara	56	280	138	142	186	94	Sugali 16	—	—	40

HH: *household*; TP: *total population*; M: *male*; F: *female*; M: *married*; UM: *unmarried*.

Table 2.2: Educational and Economic Status of the Population Studied

District	*Village*	*L*	*IL*	*Occupation*		*Land Particulars in Acres*		*Annual Income in Rupees Per HH*
				Cooli	*Agr*	*Wet*	*Dry*	
Srikakulam	Ulipiri Valasa	93	105	40	8	11	37	6191
	Ranga Puram	47	67	24	2	7	44	5023
Vizianagaram	Gandhinagar	38	44	17	4	2	40	5247
	Melikavalasa	23	32	16	16	—	32	5825
	Dippavalasa	62	71	22	6	25	60	10710
Visakhapatnam	Solabam	18	78	20	4	4	45	5666
	Modapali	130	26	32	7	22	79	9000
	Injari	27	98	20	8	10	63	6000
	Doduput	54	108	28	6	15	82	5058
	Downuru	52	40	15	3	14	62	6000
EastGodavari	I. Polavar	116	94	101	14	24	85	8000
	Kindra	72	163	110	16	27	96	6000
West Godavari	Kommu G	25	63	22	—	10	60	3000
	Vanjara	210	70	42	14	32	108	8000

L: *literate;* IL: *illiterate;* agr: *agriculture.*

inhabited by Konda Reddy and Sugali; and I. Polavaram which is inhabited by Konda Reddy and Konda Kammara. It may be noted that their literacy levels are also very basic as large majority of them attend/attended only the elementary school. With regard to their occupations large majority of them including women are found to be coolies with only a few of them who own land work on their own agricultural fields including the *podu* lands. With regard to their landholding their lands are predominantly dry lands. Their annual household incomes fall within a range of Rupees 3,000 to 10,700 with Dippavalasa village, Vizianagaram District, inhabited by Gadaba tribe recording highest average income while Kommu Gudem in West Godavari District inhabited by Koya tribe recorded the lowest with Rs. 3,000 average annual per household income.

Table 2.3 presents data related to the health status of the tribal populations covered in this study. Data related to the sick in the total village population at the time of study were collected and Kommugudem in West Godhavari District inhabited by Koya tribe with 8 out of 88 population; Gandinagar in Vizianagaram District inhabited by Jatapu and Konda Reddy Tribes with 13 out of 80 population; and Solabam in Visakhapatnam District inhabited by Porja tribe with 14 out of 96 population reported highest proportion of the sick in their population. Many sick cases are related to fever due to various etiologies including malaria. The sickness episodes were reported for during the last 15 days; one month; and two months. Visakhapatnam and East Godavari Districts reported the highest number of cases during the last 15 days at the time of this study.

From Table 2.3, it can be seen that large number of tribals in these study villages are availing the services of the Primary Health Centres. Only a few of them are still resorting to traditional medicine mostly in Visakhapatnam District with a few cases reported from East and West Godavari Districts. The local medicine men are differently called in different districts with such names like, Yejjodu, Guru, etc., is separately dealt within Chapter IV.

Table 2.4 gives an account of the health status of the mother and the child among the tribes inhabiting the Eastern Ghats based on the sample tribal villages of this study. The first column gives information related to the total number of conceptions reported in the villages studied. One still birth each in Gandhinagar in Vizianagaram, Injari and Doduput of Visakhapatnam District and

Table 2.3: Health Status of the Population Studied

District	*Village*	*Healthy Population*	*Sick*	*Sickness*		*During the Last*			*PHC*	*Tmp*
				Fever	*Other*	*15 Days*	*1 Month*	*>2 Months*		
Srikakulam	Ulipiri Valasa	189	4	4	—	4	—	—	4	—
	Ranga Puram	110	3	3	—	3	—	—	4	—
Vizianagaram	Gandhinagar	70	13	13	—	—	7	6	13	—
	Melikavalasa	55	—	—	—	—	—	—	—	—
	Dippavalasa	137	4	2	2	1	2	1	4	—
Visakhapatnam	Solabam	82	14	10	4	10	4	—	10	4
	Modapali	140	16	16		16		—	16	
	Injari	105	10	5	5	5	5	—	5	5
	Doduput	155	7	2	5	2	3	2	4	3
	Downuru	80	12	6	6	6		6	9	3
East Godavari	I. Polavar	186	24	14	10	14	4	6	20	4
	Kindra	215	20	10	10	10	5	5	20	—
West Godavari	Kommu G	80	8	4	4	4	2	2	8	—
	Vanjara	264	16	8	8	8	3	5	13	3

PHC: *Primary Health Centre;* Tmp: *Traditional Medical Practitioner.*

Table 2.4: Mother and Child Health

District	Village	Total Number of Conceptions			Reasons for Child Mortality			IFA Tablets Given during Pregnancy		How many and in what Month	
		A	B	C	D	E	F	Y	N	No. of Tablets	Month
Srikakulam	Ulipiri Valasa	12	—	—	—	—	—	12	—	100	4th
	Ranga Puram	8	—	—	—	—	—	8	—	100	4th
Vizianagaram	Gandhinagar	10	1	—	—	—	—	10	—	100	4th
	Melikavalasa	11	—	—	—	—	—	11	—	100	5th
	Dippavalasa	14	—	—	—	—	—	14	—	100	4th
Visakhapatnam	Solabam	4	—	—	—	—	—	4	—	100	4th
	Modapali	8	—	—	—	—	—	8	—	100	4th
	Injari	6	1	—	—	Low birth weight	—	4	2	100	4th
	Doduput	9	1	—	Pains	—	—	6	3	100	4th
	Downuru	4	—	—	—	—	—	4	—	100	4th
East Godavari	I.Polavar	10	—	2	—	Low birth weight	Fluid	6	2	100	4th
	Kindra	11	—	2	Pains	—	Fluid	9	—	100	4th
West Godavari	Kommu G	4	1	—	—	—	Fluid	9	—	100	4th
	Vanjara	12	—	—	—	—	—	12	—	100	4th

A: *live births;* B: *still births;* C: *abortions;* D: *severe pains;* E: *low birth weight;* F: *fluid* Y: *yes* N: *no* one in Kommugudem of West Godavari District were reported. These still births reported were due to low birth weight and fluid accumulation in the foetus. Two abortion cases each were reported from I. Polavaram and Kindra villages in East Godavari. The pregnant women were given IFA tablets in almost all cases except two cases each in Injari and I. Polavaram villages and three cases in Doduput village of Visakhapatnam District. In all the cases during the fourth month of pregnancy invariably 100 tablets were distributed.

From Table 2.5 the availing of the institutional facilities by the tribal mothers could be seen. Auxiliary Nursing Maids (ANMs) home visits were reported in the positive by all the pregnant mothers in all the villages studied except in 2 cases from I. Polavaram and one each in Kommugudem and Vanjara villages. Accordingly all the women reported to have gone to their respective PHCs to avail the facilities and counselling by the ANMS and other health workers. From Table 2.5 it can be noticed that access to the facilities of the institutional arrangements in the PHCs is available to all the tribal villagers in all the districts studied. However, only in few cases the traditional *vaid* attended to the problems related to pregnant women.

Table 2.6 gives information related to the place of delivery, who actually conducted the delivery, and whether the delivery was normal or not. It also presents data related to the use of contraceptives. In all the cases, the place of delivery was either the hospital/PHC or home. However, a large number of deliveries were reported to have taken place in the hospitals/PHCs. In large majority of the cases the medical doctor conducted the deliveries. In few other cases the deliveries were conducted by the health workers and ANMs. The deliveries were reported to be normal in all the cases except in one case in Kommugudem where there was a still birth due to accumulation of fluid. None of them reported to have used contraceptives.

Table 2.7 gives data related to immunizations given to the children of the village and the neo-natal care given by the PHC. After the delivery the umbilical cord was invariably cut by a blade and it, therefore, seems to be the usual practice among all the tribals in these districts. In all these villages the vaccinations to the infants are given for polio, diphtheria, pertussis, tetanus, measles and tuberculosis. In almost all the villages, home-based neo-natal care

Table 2.5: Mother and Child Health

District	*Village*	*During Last Pregnancy ANMs Home Visit*		*If Yes, Visit to the Health Facility*		*If No, where did you go*			
		Y	*N*	*Y*	*N*	*A*	*B*	*C*	*D*
Srikakulam	Ulipiri Valasa	12	—	12	—	—	12	—	—
	Ranga Puram	8	—	8	—	—	8	—	—
Vizianagaram	Gandhinagar	10	—	10	—	—	6	4	—
	Melikavalasa	11	—	11	—	—	6	5	—
	Dippavalasa	14	—	14	—	—	8	6	—
Visakhapatnam	Solabam	4	—	4	—	—	4	—	—
	Modapali	8	—	8	—	—	8	—	—
	Injari	6	—	6	—	—	4	2	—
	Doduput	9	—	9	—	—	6	3	—
	Downuru	4	—	4	—	—	4	—	—
East Godavari	I. Polavar	6	2	6	2	—	6	2	—
	Kindra	9		9	—	—	9	—	—
West Godavari	Kommu G	2	1	2	1	—	2	1	—
	Vanjara	12	1	12	1	—	12	—	—

A: *traditional vaid;* B: *PHC;* C: *ANM/health worker;* D: *others;* Y: *yes;* N: *no*

Table 2.6: Mother and Child Health

District	Village	Delivery was conducted at		Delivery conducted by			Weather the Delivery Normal		If, no Reasons	Used Contraceptives or not	
		A	*B*	*C*	*D*	*E*	*Y*	*N*		*Y*	*N*
Srikakulam	Ulipiri Valasa	8	4	8	2	2	12	—	—	—	12
	Ranga Puram	5	3	5	—	3	8	—	—	—	8
Vizianagaram	Gandhinagar	8	2	8	2	—	10	—	—	—	10
	Melikavalasa	6	5	6	2	3	11	—	—	—	11
	Dippavalasa	7	7	4	3	3	14	—	—	—	14
Visakhapatnam	Solabam	4	—	4	—	5	4	—	—	—	4
	Modapali	8	—	8	—	—	8	—	—	—	8
	Injari	4	2	4	—	—	6	—	—	—	6
	Doduput	6	3	6	—	2	9	—	—	—	9
	Downuru	4	—	4	—	3	4	—	—	—	4
East Godavari	I. Polavar	10	—	6	—	2	8	—	—	—	8
	Kindra	11	—	9	—	—	9	—	—	—	9
West Godavari	Kommu G	4	—	4	—	—	3	1	Fluid	—	4
	Vanjara	12	—	12	—	—	12	—	—	—	12

A: *hospital;* B: *home;* C: *doctor;* D: *ANM;* E: *health worker;* Y: *yes;* N: *no.*

Table 2.7: Mother and Child Health—Immunizations

District	Village	Object used to Cut the Umbilical Cord		Vaccinations to Infants Given for						If no, Reasons	Home Based Neo-natal Care given by PHC		Own Health Card Indicating Vaccinations Given	
		A	*B*	*C*	*D*	*E*	*F*	*G*	*H*		*Y*	*N*	*Y*	*N*
Srikakulam	Ulipiri Valasa	12	—	12	12	12	12	7	4	—	12	—	12	—
	Ranga Puram	8	—	8	8	8	8	4	3	—	8	—	8	—
Vizianagaram	Gandhinagar	10	—	10	10	10	10	5	2	—	10	—	10	—
	Melikavalasa	11	—	11	11	11	11	6	4	—	11	—	11	—
	Dippavalasa	14	—	14	14	14	14	5	-	—	14	—	14	—
Visakhapatnam	Solabam	4	—	4	4	4	4	4	1	2	4	—	4	—
	Modapali	8	—	8	8	8	8	8	4	4	8	—	8	—
	Injari	6	—	5	5	5	5	5	3	2	4	2	5	—
	Doduput	9	—	8	8	8	8	8	6	2	6	3	8	—
	Downuru	4	—	4	4	4	4	4	2	2	4	—	4	—
East Godavari	I. Polavar	8	—	8	8	8	8	8	5	3	8	—	8	—
	Kindra	9	—	9	9	9	9	9	6	3	9	—	9	—
West Godavari	Kommu G	4	—	3	3	3	3	3	1	2	4	—	3	—
	Vanjara	12	—	12	12	12	12	12	6	6	12	—	12	—

A: *blade;* C: *polio;* D: *diphtheria;* E: *pertussis;* F: *tetanus;* G: *measles;* H: *tuberculosis;* Y: *yes;* N: *no.*

was given by the PHCs except in 2 cases of Injari and 3 cases in Doduput villages of Visakhapatnam District. All the tribals of all the villages had their own health cards which indicated the vaccinations given to the children.

Table 2.8 is continuation of Immunizations experience of the tribals. The pregnant women of these tribal villages were all given tetanus toxoid injections during their ante-natal period. But hepatitis B and injectable Vi antigen were not given at all. The children between ages 12 to 23 months received vaccinations for BCG, Polio 3, DPT3, measles, and all vaccines. The children between the ages of 12 to 23 months received all the primary vaccines. Ulipirivalasa of Srikakulam District and Dippavalasa of Vizianagaram District recorded highest number of vaccinations given for polio during the last year.

Table 2.9 gives data related to nutrition among the tribals of the study villages. Children between ages of 6 to 35 months are found anaemic in all the villages studied. Although the data is in single digit in all the villages anaemia seems to be the major cause for children's morbidity in all the villages studied. Same is the case with women belonging to 15 to 49 years of age as many of them were found to be anaemic in this study. There anaemia emerges as the leading cause for the morbidity among both the mothers and the children of these tribal villages. It is found in this study that the Goitre control programme was not in operation in any of these villages. Only one case each of Goitre was reported from Ulipirivalasa of Srikakulam District, Dippavalasain of Vizianagaram District and Modapali in Visakhapatnam District. Iodized salt also was not distributed in these villages. Only one case of Vitamin A deficiency which caused corneal ulcers was reported from Gandinagar in Vizianagaram District.

Table 2.10 reflects on the performance of ICDS in these villages. Nutrition supplements like rice, dal, and oil are being supplied to the Anganwadis in these villages. It is found in this study that the performance of the ICDS was reported by the villagers as satisfactory. The tribals of the villages studied reported that the ICDS functioning in providing immunizations and ante-natal care was satisfactory except in case of 20 villagers in Ulipirivalasa in Srikakulam District and 16 in Dippavalasa of Vizianagaram District. All the tribals reported that they are having regular health check- ups except 28 in Ulipirivalasa, 26 in Rangapuram both from

Table 2.8: Immunizations

District	Village	The Pregnant Women given these during Ante-natal Period			Number of Children Received Polio Vaccine Last Year	12-23 Months Children Received the Vaccination for the Following					The Children Aged 12-23 Months Received all Primary Vaccines	
		A	B	C		D	E	F	G	H	Y	N
Srikakulam	Ulipiri Valasa	6	—	—	30	4	12	12	7	12	12	—
	Ranga Puram	9	—	—	20	3	8	8	4	8	8	—
Vizianagaram	Gandhinagar	2	—	—	15	2	10	10	5	10	10	—
	Melikavalasa	3	—	—	13	4	11	11	6	11	11	—
	Dippavalasa	5	—	—	22	—	14	14	5	14	14	—
Visakhapatnam	Solabam	4	—	—	15	2	4	4	4	4	4	—
	Modapali	8	—	—	8	4	8	8	8	8	8	—
	Injari	5	—	—	5	3	5	5	2	5	5	—
	Doduput	9	—	—	8	2	8	8	6	8	8	—
	Downuru	4	—	—	4	2	4	4	2	4	4	—
East Godavari	I. Polavar	8	—	—	8	3	8	8	5	8	8	—
	Kindra	9	—	—	9	3	9	9	6	9	9	—
West Godavari	Kommu G	3	—	—	3	2	3	3	1	3	3	—
	Vanjara	12	—	—	6	12	12	12	6	12	12	—

A: *Tetanus toxoid;* B: *hepatitis B;* C: *injectable Vi antigen typhoid vaccine;* D: *BCG;* E: *polio3;* F: *DPT3;* G: *measles;* H: *all vaccines;* Y: *Yes;* N: *no.*

Table 2.9: Nutrition

District	Village	Number of 6-35 Months Children found Anaemic	15-49 years Women found Anaemic	Goitre Control Programme in Operation or Not		Goitre Cases, if Any	Iodized Salt Supply		Vitamin-A Deficiency Reports	
				Y	N		Y	N	A	B
Srikakulam	Ulipiri Valasa	6	8	—	28	1	—	28	—	—
	Ranga Puram	7	6	—	26	—	—	26	—	—
Vizianagaram	Gandhinagar	3	4	—	19	—	—	19	1	—
	Melikavalasa	2	3	—	16	—	—	16	—	—
	Dippavalasa	4	5	—	28	1	—	28	—	—
Visakhapatnam	Solabam	6	5	—	24	—	—	24	—	—
	Modapali	4	3	—	39	1	—	39	—	—
	Injari	8	7	—	28	—	—	28	—	—
	Doduput	6	8	—	34	—	—	34	—	—
	Downuru	4	2	—	18	—	—	18	—	—
East Godavari	I. Polavar	9	11	—	42	—	—	42	—	—
	Kindra	6	8	—	47	—	—	47	—	—
West Godavari	Kommu G	7	10	—	22	—	—	22	—	—
	Vanjara	2	4	—	56	—	—	56	—	—

A: *corneal ulcers: softening of cornea;* B: *bitot spots;* Y: *yes;* N: *no.*

Table 2.10: Performance of ICDS

District	*Village*	*Nutrition Supplement Provided*			*Satisfactory Functioning of ICDS*		*ICDS Providing Immunizations, Ante-natal Care, etc.*		*Regular Health Check-ups*		*Immunizations*	
		A	*B*	*C*	*Y*	*N*	*Y*	*N*	*Y*	*N*	*Y*	*N*
Srikakulam	Ulipiri Valasa	32	32	32	32	—	28	20	—	28	28	—
	Ranga Puram	20	20	20	20	—	26	—	—	26	26	—
Vizianagaram	Gandhinagar	19	19	19	19	—	19	—	—	19	19	—
	Melikavalasa	16	16	16	16	—	16	—	16	—	16	—
	Dippavalasa	28	28	28	28	—	12	16	—	28	28	—
Visakhapatnam	Solabam	24	24	24	24	—	24	—	24	—	24	—
	Modapali	39	39	39	39	—	39	—	39	—	39	—
	Injari	28	28	28	28	—	28	—	28	—	28	—
	Doduput	34	34	34	34	—	34	—	34	—	34	—
	Downuru	18	18	18	18		18	—	18	—	18	—
East Godavari	I. Polavar	42	42	42	42	—	42	—	42	—	42	—
	Kindra	47	47	47	47	—	47	—	47	—	47	—
West Godavari	Kommu G	22	22	22	22	—	22	—	22	—	22	—
	Vanjara	56	56	56	56	—	56	—	56	—	56	

A: *rice;* B: *dal;* C: *oil;* Y: *Yes;* N: *no.*

Srikakulam District, 19 from Gandhinagar and 28 in Dippavalasa in Vizianagaram District.

Table 2.11 continues the performance of ICDS in these villages. With reference to growth promotion of the children and supplementary feeding the answer was negative invariably in all the villages. With reference to the referral services the tribal respondents seems to be not very sure as we got responses in only 6 villages with three of them answering in the positive and other three in the negative. With regard to the early childhood care of the pre-school children the tribals in all the villages except in Gandhinagar of Vizianagaram answered in the positive. The data indicate that the adolescent girls were not given any health education including nutrition. But in case of the pregnant women such health education seems to have been imparted except in case of Gandhinagar. The nursing mothers too received such an education except again in case of Gandhinagar it is in the negative.

Table 2.12 ascertains that the ICDS is working for NNAP Programme. IFA tablets were distributed to all the pregnant women by the ICDS in all the study villages. The National Vit-A PP is not in operation in any of the villages. The role of ASHA as perceived by the tribals is to distribute tablets, imparting health education and rendering assistance to the ANMs.

Table 2.13 gives an account of Prevention and Control of locally endemic diseases taken up by the health personnel as well as the villagers. DDT spraying within the house and surroundings of the house was undertaken in all the study villages in all the districts. Table 2.13 shows the number of illness episodes during the last year in the villages studied disease-wise. All the cases reported were diarrhoeal and fevers caused mostly due to malaria. The preventive and control measures taken relate to keeping the houses and surroundings clean and neat. Many of the respondents also expressed their ignorance as to the measures initiated at the village level in this regard.

Table 2.14 gives data related to the treatment of common illnesses and injuries. Large majority of the tribals in all the study villages in all the districts are availing treatment at the PHCs with a few exception of 9 in Rangapuram in Srikakulam District, 8 in Dippavalasa of Vizianagaram District, 6 in Modapali, 8 in Doduput, and 9 in Downuru in Visakhapatnam District, 7 in Kindra of East Godavari District and 4 in Kommugudem of West Godavari District

Table 2.11: Performance of ICDS

District	Village	Growth Promotion and Supplementary Feeding		Referral Services Provided		Early Childhood Care and Pre-school Education		Nutrition and Health Education Given for Adolescent Girls		Nutrition and Health Education for Pregnant Women		Nutrition and Health Education to Nursing Mothers	
		Y	N	Y	N	Y	N	Y	N	Y	N	Y	N
Srikakulam	Ulipiri Valasa	—	28	20	8	28	—	—	28	28	—	28	—
	Ranga Puram	—	26	—	26	26	—	—	26	26	—	26	—
Vizianagaram	Gandhinagar	—	19	—	19	—	19	—	19	—	19	—	19
	Melikavalasa	—	16	16	—	16	—	—	16	16	—	16	—
	Dippavalasa	—	28	28	—	28	—	—	28	28	—	28	—
Visakhapatnam	Solabam	—	24	—	—	24	—	—	24	24	—	24	—
	Modapali	—	39	—	—	39	—	—	39	39	—	39	—
	Injari	—	28	—	—	28	—	—	28	28	—	28	—
	Doduput	—	34	—	—	34	—	—	34	34	—	34	—
	Downuru	—	18	—	—	18	—	—	18	18	—	18	—
East Godavari	I. Polavar	—	42	—	—	42	—	—	42	42	—	42	—
	Kindra	—	47	—	—	47	—	—	47	47	—	47	—
West Godavari	Kommu G	—	22	—	—	22	—	—	22	22	—	22	—
	Vanjara	—	56	—	—	56	—	—	56	56	—	56	—

Y: *yes;* N: *no.*

Table 2.12: Performance of ICDS

District	Village	Working for NNAP Programme		IFA Supplied for Pregnant Women		How many Days	Do You Work for N.Vit-A PP		Role of ASHA		
		Y	N	Y	N	100	Y	N	A	B	C
Srikakulam	Ulipiri Valasa	28	—	28	—	100	—	48	48	48	—
	Ranga Puram	26	—	26	—	100	—	26	26	26	—
Vizianagaram	Gandhinagar	19	—	19	—	100	—	19	19	—	—
	Melikavalasa	16	—	16	—	100	—	16	16	16	16
	Dippavalasa	28	—	28	—	100	—	28	28	28	28
Visakhapatnam	Solabam	24	—	24	—	100	—	24	24	24	—
	Modapali	39	—	39	—	100	—	39	39	39	—
	Injari	28	—	28	—	100	—	28	28	28	—
	Doduput	34	—	34	—	100	—	34	34	34	—
	Downuru	18	—	18	—	100	—	18	18	18	—
East Godavari	I. Polavar	42	—	42	—	100	—	42	42	42	—
	Kindra	47	—	47		100	—	47	47	47	—
West Godavari	Kommu G	22	—	22	—	100	—	22	22	22	—
	Vanjara	56	—	56	—	100	—	56	56	56	—

A: *tablets distribution;* B: *assistance to ANM;* C: *health education;* Y: *yes* N: *no.*

Table 2.13: Prevention and Control of Locally Endemic Diseases

District	*Village*	*Indoor Residual Spraying with DDT Surrounding the House*		*Number of Cases Reported in the Family during the Last Year for the following*								*Prevention and Control Measures Taken for Each of the Above*	
		Y	*N*	*A*	*B*	*C*	*D*	*E*	*F*	*G*	*H*	*I*	*J*
Srikakulam	Ulipiri Valasa	48	—	—	20	15	—	—	—	—	—	22	26
	Ranga Puram	26	—	—	14	18	—	—	—	—	—	14	12
Vizianagaram	Gandhinagar	19	—	—	2	4	—	—	—	—	—	16	3
	Melikavalasa	16	—	—	4	5	—	—	—	—	—	9	7
	Dippavalasa	28	—	—	8	12	—	—	—	—	—	15	13
Visakhapatnam	Solabam	24	—	—	6	12	—	—	—	—	—	12	12
	Modapali	39	—	—	4	5	—	—	—	—	—	15	24
	Injari	28	—	—	12	8	—	—	—	—	—	17	11
	Doduput	34	—	—	5	4	—	—	—	—	—	16	18
	Downuru	18	—	—	6	7	—	—	—	—	—	9	9
East Godavari	I. Polavar	42	—	—	11	14	—	—	—	—	—	20	22
	Kindra	47	—	—	5	10	—	—	—	—	—	30	17
West Godavari	Kommu G	22	—	—	4	2	—	—	—	—	—	12	10
	Vanjara	56	—	—	8	12	—	—	—	—	—	36	20

A: *HIV/AIDS;* B: *diarrhoeal;* C: *malaria;* D: *radesh;* E: *Japanese encephalitis;* F: *dengue;* G: *chickun gunya;* H: *leprosy;* I: *maintain neatness;* J: *do not know;* Y: *yes;* N: *no.*

Table 2.14: Treatment of Common Illnesses and Injuries

District	*Village*	*Where do you go for Treatment*			*What Ailments do you consult him*		*Fees Particulars*	*Method of Treatment*
		A	*B*	*C*	*D*	*E*		*Mantram*
Srikakulam	Ulipiri Valasa	48	—	—	—	—	—	—
	Ranga Puram	17	9	—	fever	pain	—	9
Vizianagaram	Gandhinagar	19	—	—	—	—	—	—
	Melikavalasa	16	—	—	—	—	hen/Rs. 10	—
	Dippavalasa	20	8	—	8	—	—	8
Visakhapatnam	Solabam	18		—	—	—	—	Mantram
	Modapali	39	6	—	—	—	—	—
	Injari	20		—	—	—	—	—
	Doduput	25	8	—	—	—	—	—
	Downuru	18	9	—	—	—	—	—
East Godavari	I. Polavar	42		—	—	—	—	—
	Kindra	40	7	—	—	—	—	—
West Godavari	Kommu G	18	4	—	—	—	—	—
	Vanjara	56		—	—	—	—	—

A: *PHC;* B: *traditional healer;* C: *guruvu;* D: *fever;* E: *pain.*

were to be still using the services of the local traditional healers. The local medicine man/shaman is usually consulted for fevers and body pains for a fee of a hen and Rupees 10/-. The usual method of treatment followed by them in most cases is chanting of *mantra* (incantations). A separate chapter in this report deals with the local medicine men/shaman.

Table 2.15 is the continuation of Table 2.14. PHC Doctor is mostly preferred by all the tribals in all the villages of all the districts. A few of them 9 from Rangapuram, 8 from Dippavalasa, 6 from Solabam, 8 from Injari, 9 from Doduput, 7 from Kindra and 4 from Kommugudem preferred ANMs. This preference of ANMs is mostly due to the long absence of the PHC Doctor. As in many PHCs it is observed Doctors go on long leave leaving the posts lying vacant for a long time. With regard to the services the tribals are receiving from ASHA of the responses relate to receiving of tablets and health education. Except in Doduput village in Visakhapatnam in all the other villages there is the presence of ASHA. Although a few of the villagers answered in the negative it has to be considered as their ignorance of such a person ASHA. With regard to the performance of ASHA, a large majority of the tribal villagers expressed satisfaction. Only a few of them answered in the negative.

Table 2.16 is the continuation of Tables 2.14 and 2.15. A little more dedication and responsibility is found wanting according to many tribal respondents in addition to have more health education from her. With regard to ASHAs training in dealing with the generic diseases the responses invariably were in the negative. Mothers seem to have been given orientation in using ORS solution. There is no such thing as school sanitation in all the villages studied except in Modapali and Doduput in Visakhapatnam District in Kindra and Vanjara of East and West Godavari Districts respectively.

Table 2.17 deals with water supply and sanitation. No technological improvisations introduced in all the study villages but IEC (information, education and communication) campaigns were undertaken in all these villages. With regard to any one trying to bring about any behavioural changes among them the reply was in negative by all the tribals of this study. As to their awareness of Nirmal Gram Puraskar the answer mostly was in the negative except in case of 30 tribals in Modapali,20 in Doduput in Visakhapatnam district, 20 in I. Polavaram and 39 in Kindra of

Table 2.15: Treatment of Common Illnesses and Injuries

District	*Village*	*Whom do You prefer among the Other Medical Practitioners*			*What Services do you receive from ASHA*		*Are you satisfied with her Performance*		*Presence of ASHA in your village*	
		A	*B*	*C*	*D*	*E*	*Y*	*N*	*Y*	*N*
Srikakulam	Ulipiri Valasa	48	—	—	30	18	35	13	40	8
	Ranga Puram	17	9	—	16	10	16	10	16	10
Vizianagaram	Gandhinagar	19	—	—	19	—	19	—	19	—
	Melikavalasa	16	—	—	16	16	11	5	16	—
	Dippavalasa	20	8	—	—	28	28	—	20	8
Visakhapatnam	Solabam	18	6	—	16	8	18	4	16	8
	Modapali	39	—	—	39	—	39	—	39	—
	Injari	20	8	—	20	8	20	8	20	8
	Doduput	25	9	—	20	14	20	14	—	34
	Downuru	18	—	—	18	18	9	9	18	—
East Godavari	I. Polavar	42	—	—	42	42	42	—	42	—
	Kindra	40	7	—	20	27	47	—	40	7
West Godavari	Kommu G	18	4	—	16	6	15	7	18	4
	Vanjara	56	—	—	56	56	56	—	56	—

A: *PHC doctor;* B: *ANM;* C: *traditional healer;* D: *receives tablets;* E: *health education;* Y: *yes;* N: *no.*

Table 2.16: Treatment of Common Illnesses and Injuries

District	*Village*	*What else do you expect from ASHA*			*Mothers Orientation to use ORS Solution*		*ASHA got trained to deal with Generic Ailments at Village*		*If Yes what kind*		*Any such things as School Sanitation*	
		A	*B*	*C*	*Y*	*N*	*Y*	*N*	*Y*	*N*	*Y*	*N*
Srikakulam	Ulipiri Valasa	—	—	—	48	—	—	48	—	48	—	48
	Ranga Puram	—	—	—	26	—	—	26	—	26	—	26
Vizianagaram	Gandhinagar	—	—	—	19	—	—	19	4	15	—	19
	Melikavalasa	—	—	—	16	—	—	16	—	16	—	16
	Dippavalasa	—	—	—	24	4	—	28	—	28	—	28
Visakhapatnam	Solabam		—	—	24	—	—	24	—	24	—	24
	Modapali	—	—	—	39	—	—	—	39	—	39	—
	Injari	—	—	—	21	7	—	28	—	—	—	—
	Doduput	—	—	—	34	—	—	34	34	—	34	—
	Downuru	—	—	—	10	8	—	18	—	18	—	18
East Godavari	I. Polavar	—	—	—	42	—	—	42	—	42	—	42
	Kindra	—	—	—	40	7	—	47	47	—	47	—
West Godavari	Kommu G	15	7	—	15	7		22	—	22		22
	Vanjara	56	—	—	40	16		56	56		56	

A: *dedication;* B: *need more health knowledge;* C: *responsibility;* Y: *yes;* N: *no.*

Table 2.17: Water Supply, Sanitation and Health Education

District	Village	Any Technological Improvisation		IEC Campaign		Anyone tried to bring about Relevant Behavioural Changes		Aware of Nirmal Gram Puraskar		How often do you clean your Teeth and Body		
		Y	N	Y	N	Y	N	Y	N	A	B	C
Srikakulam	Ulipiri Valasa	—	48	48	—	—	48	—	48	20	10	18
	Ranga Puram	—	26	26	—	—	26	—	26	15	8	3
Vizianagaram	Gandhinagar	—	19	19	—	—	19	—	19	9	4	6
	Melikavalasa	—	16	16	—	—	16	—	16	10	3	3
	Dippavalasa	—	28	28	—	—	28	—	28	18	6	4
Visakhapatnam	Solabam	—	24	24	—	—	24	—	24	18	—	—
	Modapali	—	—	—	—	—	—	30	9	29	5	5
	Injari	—	—	—	—	—	—	—	28	20	8	—
	Doduput	—	34	34	—	—	—	20	14	20	14	—
	Downuru	—	18	18	—	—	18	—	18	10	8	—
East Godavari	I. Polavar	—	42	42	—	—	42	20	22	20	8	14
	Kindra	—	47	47	—	—	47	39	8	15	15	17
West Godavari	Kommu G	—	22	22	—	—	22	—	22	12	10	—
	Vanjara	—	56	56	—	—	56	56	—	20	5	31

A: *once in a day*; B: *once in two days*; C: *once in three days*; Y: *yes;* N: *no.*

East Godavari Districts and 56 in Vanjara of West Godavari District. With regard to their personal cleanliness related to cleaning of teeth, about one-fourth of the households reported once in three days and another one-fourth once in two days. Only half of them reported it as once daily. Vanjara in East Godavari, Ulipirivalasa in Srikakulam District, I. Polavaram and Kindra in East Godavari Districts reported large number of tribals cleaning their teeth once in three days.

Table 2.18 is the continuation of the topic on Health Education. With regard to how often they change clothes about half of them reported it as in three days and the remaining half in five days. This partly reflects on their economic status. Large majority of them were found to be washing their clothes in the stream water and the rest of them using the well water or hand pump. The major sources of potable water for these tribals are the well, the bore well and the stream in the study villages still 40 per cent of them are using stream for their drinking purpose. As water borne diseases among the tribals constitute highest proportion their etiology could be traced to such a practice of consuming the stream water. Boiling water before consumption was reported in the negative by all the tribals of this study. Of course boiling requires more firewood which could be another problem for most of the tribals. About 36 per cent tribal households of the present study reported not using soap to wash their bodies probably due to their poverty.

Table 2.19 is the continuation of data on health education. A large majority of the tribals are found using fire wood for cooking purpose. Only a few of them are using cooking gas and majority of them are from West Godavari District, 22 households (100%) from Kommugudem and 16 are from Vanjara. The rest are from Kindra from East Godavari, Downuru and Modapali from Visakhapatnam District. The food is reported to have been undercooked many a time which could be a cause for their ill health. Defecation by the tribals is mostly on the road side with a few exceptions of using the latrines as in case of 20 in Vanjira, 15 in Kindra, 10 in Dippavalasa. Washing hands thoroughly after defecation also was reported in the negative by all the tribals. Not a single HIV/AIDS case was reported by this study sample.

Table 2.20 gives information related to episodes of sickness. Large majority of the tribals expressed the need for more number

Table 2.18: Health Education

District	Village	How often do you change clothes		Where do you wash clothes			Source of Potable Water			Boiling of the Water for Drinking		Do you use soap	
		A	B	C	D	E	F	G	H	Y	N	Y	N
Srikakulam	Ulipiri Valasa	28	20	—	28	20	28	20	—	—	48	30	18
	Ranga Puram	10	16	—	—	26	10	10	6	—	26	20	6
Vizianagaram	Gandhinagar	7	12	12	7	—	12	7	—	—	19	14	5
	Melikavalasa	7	8	—	—	16	16	—	—	—	16	10	6
	Dippavalasa	10	18	—	—	28	20	8	—	—	28	20	8
Visakhapatnam	Solabam	9	9	—	—	18	10	—	10	—	18	10	8
	Modapali	20	19	12	10	17	—	—	39	—	39	29	10
	Injari	8	20	—	—	28	—	—	28	—	28	10	18
	Doduput	4	30	—	—	34	—	—	34	—	34	10	24
	Downuru	8	10	8	10	—	8	10	—	—	18	15	3
East Godavari	I. Polavar	30	12	—	—	42	10	12	20	—	42	27	20
	Kindra	29	13	10	15	22	12	15	20	—	47	32	15
West Godavari	Kommu G	4	18	—	—	22	—	—	22	—	22	15	7
	Vanjara	40	16	30	16	—	15	20	21	—	56	40	16

A: *once in three days;* B: *once in five days;* C: *well;* D: *hand pump;* E: *stream;* F: *well* G: *hand pump;* H: *stream;* Y: *yes;* N: *no*

Table 2.19: Health Education

District	Village	How the food is cooked		Is it well cooked always		Where do you defecate		Role of Mass Media		Washing of hands thoroughly		HIV and Other Lifestyle Diseases	
		A	B	C	D	E	F	G	H	Y	N	Y	N
Srikakulam	Ulipiri Valasa	48	—	—	48	—	48	—	—	—	48	—	48
	Ranga Puram	26	—	—	26	—	26	—	—	—	26	—	26
Vizianagaram	Gandhinagar	19	—	—	19	—	19	—	—	—	19	—	19
	Melikavalasa	16	—	—	16	—	16	4	12	—	16	—	16
	Dippavalasa	28	—	—	28	10	38	—	—	—	28	—	28
Visakhapatnam	Solabam	18	—	—	18	—	18	—	—	—	24	—	24
	Modapali	34	5	—	39	6	33	—	—	—	39	—	39
	Injari	28	—	—	28	—	28	—	—	—	28	—	28
	Doduput	34	—	—	34	6	34	—	—	—	34	—	34
	Downuru	11	7	—	18	—	18	—	—	—	18	—	18
East Godavari	I. Polavar	42	—	—	42	7	35	—	—	—	42	—	42
	Kindra	40	7		47	15	32	—	—	—	47	—	47
West Godavari	Kommu G	—	22	—	22	—	22	—	—	—	22	—	22
	Vanjara	40	16	—	56	20	36	—	—	—	56	—	56

A: *fire wood;* B: *gas;* C: *well cooked;* D: *under cooked;* E: *latrine;* F: *road side;* G: *good;* H: *don't know;* Y: *yes;* N: no.

Table 2.20: Episodes of Sickness

District	Village	Contextual Needs			Who diagnosed		Sickness during Last Year		Mortalities during Last Year		Recent Health Campaign conducted		Health Melas conducted		Sickness during Last Month	
		A	B	C	D	E	Y	N	Y	N	Y	N	Y	N	Y	N
Srikakulam	Ulipiri Valasa	48	—	—	22	—	29	—	—	48	—	—	—	—	22	—
	Rangapuram	26	—	—	10	5	20	—	2	24	—	26	—	26	15	—
Vizianagaram	Gandhinagar	—	—	—	14	—	13	6	—	19	—	19	—	19	14	5
	Melikavalasa	4	10	2	4	—	14	2	—	16	16	—	—	16	4	12
	Dippavalasa	—	—	—	28	—	20	—	—	28	—	28	—	28	17	11
Visakhapatnam	Solabam	24	—	—	12	—	15	—	—	24	—	—	—	24	12	—
	Modapali	39	—	—	10	—	18	—	—	39	39	—	39	—	10	—
	Injari	—	—	—	9	—	7	—	—	28	—	28	—	28	9	—
	Doduput	—	—	—	10	—	12	—	1	33	34	—	—	34	10	—
	Downuru	—	—	—	7	—	8	—	—	18	—	—	—	—	7	—
East Godavari	I. Polavar	—	—	—	12	—	17	—	—	42	42	—	—	42	12	
	Kindra	—	—	—	14	—	20	—	—	47	—	—	—		14	
West Godavari	Kommu G	—	—	—	8	—	12	—	—	22	—	—	—	—	8	—
	Vanjara	—	—	—	12	—	17	—	—	56	56	—	—	56	12	—

A: *staff;* B: *communication facilities;* C: *staff stayed in head quarters;* D: *PHC doctor* E: *traditional healer* Y: *yes;* N: *no.*

of health professionals posted in their areas. Very few of the health staff are staying in the quarters for varied reasons. Many of them also expressed that the communication facilities in their areas must be improved. During the last year sickness was reported in all the households with 2 mortalities in Rangapuram of Srikakulam District and one in Doduput village of Visakhapatnam District. Health campaigns were reported in 5 of the villages studied and except in Modapali in no other village health *melas* were conducted. During the last month of the study except in a few households in three villages all the households in all the villages in all the Districts sickness was reported.

Inter-Tribal Differences

With respect to sickness episodes the Porja tribe, a primitive tribe is at the top. It may be noted that other primitive tribes like the Kondhs, Gadabas and the Savaras too suffer more than other tribes (Subramanyam, 2007: 28-44). One still birth each was reported from Kondu, Gadaba, Koya and Jatapu tribes. Kondu and Gadaba are the primitive tribes (Table 2.4). In case of deliveries conducted Gadabas, Jatapus, Kondu and Savaras recorded more number of deliveries as done at home. A Koya woman reported accumulation of fluid in the womb (Table 2.6). The Nutritional status reflected in Table 2.9 does not reflect any remarkable differences among the different tribal groups as all of them by and large were found to be anaemic. The traditional healer (shaman) still treating the sick is found more among the Savaras, Valmikis, Gadaba, Kondu, in that order. With the exception of Valmikis all others are primitive tribal groups. It may be noted here that many of them preferred the ANM to the PHC Doctor probably because of their intimacy with the ANMs (Table 2.15). Many Savaras and Kondhs expressed ignorance as to the presence of ASHA in their village. More number of Valmikis and Sugalis reported cleaning their teeth once in two/three days compared to other tribes Table (2.17). Two deaths among the Savaras and one in Kondu tribe during the last year were reported in our study sample (Table 2.20). Both the tribes are classified as primitive tribes.

III
PHCs Role in Tribal Primary Health Care

Ever since the Family Planning Programmes were introduced in 1952, India has progressed remarkably in areas related to maternal and child health. For example, according to the 2005 National Family Health survey, total fertility rate is brought down from 6 to 2.9; Maternal mortality ratio to 301 SRS per 100,000 live births; infant mortality rate from 146 to 58; child mortality rate (0-4) from 57.3 to 17 (NFHS-3-2005-06). However, the situation related to tribals in this area still needs to be improved. Table 3.1 presents the maternal illnesses and the available obstetric services in the PHCs studied in the nine districts of Andhra Pradesh.

Among the methods adopted for the promotion of contraceptives use, distribution of condoms and use of Copper-T and oral pills in cases of tubectomy are found to be the usual methods practiced in all the PHCs with East Godavary District in the lead probably because of the high incidence of HIV/AIDS in that district. Distribution of condoms by the PHCs is found in all the PHCs of all the districts but the distribution of IEC material and advices related to spacing methods are found to be given not much importance in all the PHCs except in two or three districts (East and West Godavari and Visakhapatnam Districts) reflecting the poor performance of the PHCs staff in this area. Obstructed labour and hypertensive disorders are predominant of all the maternal illnesses reported in this study. The highest incidence of these cases was reported from Khammam District followed by Vizianagaram. Haemorrhage, sepsis and abortions constitute

Table 3.1: Mother and Child Health: Illnesses, Anti-Natal Checkups of Obstetric Services

S. No.	District	Methods adopted for Contraceptives Promotion			Cases related to (during the last year) Various Illnesses					Anti-natal Check-ups during Last Year			Essential Obstetric Services provided										Supply of Contraceptives by PHC/Sub-centre	
		A	B	C	D	E	F	G	H	I	J	K	L	M	N	O	P	Q	R	S	T	U	Y	N
1.	SK	-	-	4	3	3	7	17	15	656	96	752	4	4	4	3	4	-	-	2361	4	-	4	-
2.	VZ	-	-	4	-	-	-	454	-	1573	607	2180	4	4	4	4	4	-	-	1100	4	-	4	-
3.	VS	11	4	2		2	12			12350	4109	16459	11	11	2	4	8			7500	9	2	11	-
4.	EG	14	14	10	-	-	13			1651	545	2202	14	14	8	2	10			7000	10	4	14	-
5.	WG	-	6	6	-	-	-	-	5	1350	250	1600	6	6	6	3	3	-	-	4044	6	-	6	-
6.	KA	-	-	5	-	16	13	320	1681	2000	337	2337	5	5	5	5	5	-	-	4950	5	-	5	-
7.	NL	-	-	3	-	-	-	4	-	1477	250	1727	3	3	3	3	3	-	-	2560	3	-	3	-
8.	MN	-	-	2	3	-	10	2	10	250	150	400	2	2	2	2	2	-	-	240	2	-	2	-
9.	CU	-	-	2	2	-	6	-	156	1810	368	2178	2	2	2	2	2	-	-	1784	2	-	2	-

SK: *Srikakulam*; VZ: *Vizianagaram*; VS: *Visakhapatnam*; EG: *East Godavari*; WG: *West Godavari*; KA: *Khammam*; NL: *Nellore*; MN: *Mahaboobnagar*; CU: *Cuddapah*; A: *spacing method*; B: *IEC material*; C: *condom, Copper-T, tubectomy*; D: *hemorrhage*; E: *sepsis*; F: *Abortion*; G: *Obstructed labour*; H: *hypertensive disorder*; I: *PHC*; J: *home*; K: *total*; L: *antenatal care*; M: *Institutional safe delivery practices*; N: *postnatal care for early and timely detection of emergencies*; O: *provision of 24 hours delivery services at all CHCs and PHCs*; P: *postnatal care for mothers and new born*; Q: *what kinds of injections are given (specify)*; R: *what are the interventions initiated to save the mother and child*; S: *how many institutional deliveries during the last five years*; T: *deliveries conducted by trained personnel in domiciliary delivery*; U: *deliveries conducted by untrained personnel.*

insignificant proportion. Anti-natal check ups are done by all the PHCs in all the districts both at home and in the PHCs as per the data but the authenticity of it is doubtful. However, these figures could be taken as indicative of the PHCs awareness to such a performance (Table 3.1). Deliveries were done in the PHCs in all the districts within a range of 48-1500 per annum with Visakhapatnam leading the figures because of the high concentration of tribals. Other obstetric services provided are the provision of 24 hours delivery services, post-natal care for mothers and the new born. The injections that were used and the interventions to save the mother and child were not provided by any of the PHCs. A few deliveries conducted by untrained persons were reported from the PHCs of Visakhapatnam and East Godavari districts.

Some of the important causes of maternal mortality in India are as follows:

Haemorrhage—38 per cent; Sepsis—11 per cent; abortion—8 per cent; obstructed labour—5 per cent; hypertensive disorders—5 per cent; other conditions—34 per cent.

Emergency obstetric care and safe abortion facilities ensure the survival and health of the mother and the child. Table 3.2 gives data related to these practices and the presence of Accredited Social Health Activist in the villages under these PHCs. In almost all the PHCs studied in all the district referral services are found to be available except in the case of one PHC in Visakhapatnam, two in West Godavari, three in East Godavari and five in Khammam District. But in large majority of First Referral Units (FRUs) blood storage facility is absent. It is also found that in many cases the doctors who man these PHCs do not have training in life-saving anesthetic skills and emergency obstetric management care. Although abortions are done under medical supervision and there are almost an equal number of them without adequate medical supervision. Provision of quality manual vacuum aspiration facility is absent in all the PHCs except in case of two PHCs in Vizianagaram and one each in Nalgonda and Cuddapah.

Child Health

The infant mortality rate (IMR) in 2005 is 58 per 1000 live births (SRS, RGI Office). It is lower in urban areas at 40/1000 live births than in rural areas which is 64/1000 live births. Although accurate information on tribal is not available, it is the highest our country

Table 3.2: Mother and Child Health: Obstetric Care and ASHA

S. No.	District	Emergency Obstetric Care at FRU								Safe Abortion Facilities				Presence of ASHA	
		A		B		C		D		E		F		Y	N
		Y	N	Y	N	Y	N	Y	N	Y	N	Y	N		
1.	SK	4	-	1	3	-	4	-	4	2	2	-	4	199	120
2.	VZ	4	-	-	4	-	4	4	-	2	2	2	2	220	87
3.	VS	10	1	2	11	7	4	4	7	11	-	-	11	1265	460
4.	EG	11	3	7	7	10	4	8	6	7	7	-	14	401	125
5.	WG	4	2	3	3	6	-	4	2	-	6	-	6	263	45
6.	KA	-	5	-	5	-	5	3	2	5	-	-	5	263	18
7.	NL	3	-	-	3	-	3	-	3	1	2	1	2	182	28
8.	MN	2	-	-	2	1	1	1	1	1	1	-	2	6	1
9.	CU	2	-	-	2	1	1	1	1	2	-	1	1	136	-

SK: *Srikakulam;* VZ: *Vizianagaram;* VS: *Visakhapatnam;* EG: *East Godavari;* WG: *West Godavari;* KA: *Khammam;* NL: *Nellore;* MN: *Mahaboobnagar;* CU: *Cuddapah;* A: *what referral services at community and institutional levels are available;* B: *is there a blood storage centre at FRUs;* C: *have the MBBS doctors got trained in life-saving anesthetic skills for emergency obstetric care;* D: *have the MBBS doctors got trained in emergency obstetric management skills;* E: *medical abortion under medical supervision;* F: *provision of quality manual vacuum aspiration facility at the PHC.*

has ever recorded. Table 3.3 presents the incidence of IMR, Neo-natal deaths and the most frequent causes of ill health among the children. Table 3.3 also presents the measures taken by the PHC/ ICDS to promote breast/complementary feeding in areas related to the PHCs in all the districts of this study.

From Table 3.3, it can be seen that higher IMRs are reported from the three north coastal Andhra Districts of Srikakulam, Vizianagaram and Visakhapatnam Districts. The causes are poor hygienic conditions at the PHCs, low birth weight and malnutrition. Number of children who were ill during the last year is also shown in the table. Diarrhoea is the major cause and the highest number of cases is reported from Khammam District followed by Vizianagaram and Nellore Districts. Water contamination and insufficient availability of potable water in these areas could be the reasons for such high incidence. Malaria accounts for another major cause that contributes to child

Table 3.3: Child Health: Mortality and Feeding Practices

S. No.	District	Prevalence of Infant Mortality			Cases related to during Last Year				Neo-natal Deaths (pre-maturity, Sepsis)		Measures taken to promote Breast Feeding		Measures taken to promote complementary Feeding		
		A	*B*	*C*	*D*	*E*	*F*	*G*	*H*	*I*	*J*	*K*	*L*	*M*	*N*
1.	SK	—	—	24	—	—	24	14	3	2	—	4	—	—	4
2.	VZ	4	3	15	789	—	232	537	15	—	4	3	4	4	—
3.	VS	10	11	4	305	—	275	—	14	—	11	—	10	9	—
4.	EG	8	4	2	240	—	185	2	—	—	10	4	8	8	4
5.	WG	4	2	—	10	—	235	—	—	—	4	2	5	1	—
6.	KA	—	5	—	2148	6	718	163	3	—	—	—	—	—	—
7.	NL	—	—	2	561	—	360	119	—	—	—	—	—	—	—
8.	MN	—	—	2	200	3	20	5	—	—	—	2	2	—	—
9.	CU	—	—	—	178	2	47	36	5	—	—	—	2	—	—

SK: *Srikakulam;* VZ: *Vizianagaram;* VS: *Visakhapatnam;* EG: *East Godavari;* WG: *West Godavari;* KA: *Khammam;* NL: *Nellore;* MN: *Mahaboobnagar;* CU: *Cuddapah;* A: *low birth weight;* B: *malnutrition;* C: *poor hygienic conditions;* D: *diarrhoea;* E: *measles;* F: *malaria;* G: *malnutrition;* H: *pre-maturity;* I: *sepsis;* J: *immunity power;* K: *health education;* L: *immunity power;* M: *more nutrients;* N: *health education.*

mortalities and morbidities. Vizianagaram, Khammam and Nellore Districts registered more number of such cases of malaria. The overall neo-natal deaths are very small in number and the few cases reported are due to pre-mature deliveries and sepsis.

Imparting of health education to improve the general immunity of the mother and the child are the measures taken by the PHCs to promote the breast feeding of the child by the mothers. More nutritious food in addition to health education are some of the measures taken by the ICDS to promote complementary feeding. It may be noted here that malnutrition has not declined significantly over the last decade: it was 54 per cent in 92-93; 47 per cent in 98-99; 46 per cent in 2005-06.

In case of neo-natal mortality, Integrated Management of Neo-natal and Childhood Illnesses (IMNCI) was the major initiative under the Reproductive Child Health Programme. This strategy includes a range of interventions to prevent and manage five major childhood illnesses such as ARI, diarrhoea, measles, malaria, and malnutrition. The major components of this strategy include, the strengthening the skills of health care workers, strengthening the health care infrastructure and the involvement of the community. Table 3.4 shows the performance of the PHCs/ ICDS in this context.

It is interesting to notice that all the PHCs studied reported undertaking of the strengthening of skills of their health care workers. The involvement of the community which is very crucial to improve the health standards of the people was reported in all the PHCs except in Srikakulam district where four PHCs reported in the negative. In case of Anti-malarial programmes too the district reported in the negative. Home-based neo-natal care was reported from all the PHCs except three in Vizianagaram and 2 in Visakhapatnam. The training of the ANMs is a mixed bag as large number of them, 20 from Srikakulam and 10 from Vizianagaram Districts reported in the negative. In other districts a small number of them reported positively.

The National Health Policy (1983) accorded high priority to the immunization of children, and universal immunization against the six vaccine preventable diseases (VPD). Pulse polio immunization was initiated in 1994.

From Table 3.5 it can be seen that all the PHCs have administered the vaccinations for polio, diphtheria, pertussis,

Table 3.4: Child Health: ICDS, ANMS, and their Skills

S. No.	District	Strengthening Skills of Health Care Workers		Strengthening of Health Care Infrastructure		Involvement of Community		Performance of ICDS		Anti-Malarial Programmes		Home based Neo-natal Care		ANMs got Trained in RAI	
		Y	N	Y	N	Y	N	Y	N	Y	N	Y	N	Y	N
1.	Srikakulam	9	—	11	—	7	4	9	2	—	11	11	—	—	20
2.	Vizianagaram	14	—	14	—	14	—	12	2	14	—	11	3	4	10
3.	Visakhapatnam	6	—	6	—	6	—	6	—	6	—	4	2	—	6
4.	East Godavari	4	—	4	—	4	—	4	—	4	—	4	—	3	1
5.	West Godavari	4	—	4	—	4	—	4	—	4	—	4	—	2	2
6.	Khammam	1	—	3	—	3	—	3	—	3	—	3	—	3	—
7.	Nellore	5	—	5	—	5	—	5	—	5	—	5	—	5	—
8.	Mahboobnagar	2	—	2	—	2	—	2	—	2	—	2	—	1	1
9.	Cuddapah	2	—	2	—	2	—	2	—	2	—	2	—	1	1

Y: yes; N: no.

Table 3.5: Immunization: Various Vaccinations

S. No.	District	Vaccinations to Infants given for												Pregnant Women Vaccination		12-23 Months received Vaccinations	
		A		B		C		D		E		F		TT	Other		
		Y	N	Y	N	Y	N	Y	N	Y	N	Y	N			Y	N
1.	SK	4	—	4	—	4	—	4	—	4	—	4	—	4	—	4	—
2.	VZ	4	—	4	—	4	—	4	—	4	—	4	—	4	—	4	—
3.	VS	11	—	11	—	11	—	11	—	11	—	11	—	11	—	7	4
4.	EG	14	—	14	—	14	—	14	—	14	—	14	—	14	—	10	4
5.	WG	6	—	6	—	6	—	6	—	6	—	6	—	6	—	6	—
6.	KA	5	—	5	—	5	—	5	—	5	—	5	—	5	—	5	—
7.	NL	3	—	3	—	3	—	3	—	3	—	3	—	3	—	3	—
8.	MN	2	—	2	—	2	—	2	—	2	—	2	—	2	—	2	—
9.	CU	2	—	2	—	2	—	2	—	2	—	2	—	2	—	2	—

SK: *Srikakulam*; VZ: *Vizianagaram*; VS: *Visakhapatnam*; EG: *East Godavari*; WG: *West Godavari*; KA: *Khammam*; NL: *Nellore*; MN: *Mahaboobnagar*; CU: *Cuddapah*; A: *polio*; B: *diphtheria*; C: *pertussis*; D: *tetanus*; E: *measles*; F: *tuberculosis*; G: TT (*Tetanus Toxoid*); H: *other*.

measles and tuberculosis. The pregnant women invariably are given Tetanus toxoid injections and the babies between 12 and 23 months old were administered vaccines.

Table 3.5.1 presents the total number of vaccinations given in the PHCs studies in all the districts covered under Eastern Ghats. Administration of Polio vaccine seems to be very successful in all the PHCs.

Table 3.5.1: Vaccinations

S. No.	*District*	*Polio Vaccine*	*12-23 Months received Vaccinations for the following*				
			A	*B*	*C*	*D*	*E*
1.	SR	5690	922	1391	1391	1407	2690
2.	VM	5967	860	994	919	888	2875
3.	VS	14172	2171	2864	2940	1665	4670
4.	EG	12152	2019	2796	2563	1549	4458
5.	WG	8893	2955	2955	3111	1773	3656
6.	KA	6555	160	160	158	158	200
7.	NL	7262	—	—	—	—	—
8.	MN	1990	345	340	340	330	330
9.	CU	9862	145	145	145	110	560

SK: *Srikakulam;* VZ: *Vizianagaram;* VS: *Visakhapatnam;* EG: *East Godavari;* WG: *West Godavari;* KA: *Khammam;* NL: Nellore; MN: *Mahaboobnagar;* CU: *Cuddapah;* A: *BCG;* B: *Polio;* C: *DPT;* D: *Measles;* E: *All Vaccines.*

Table 3.6 presents the nutritional status of the tribals from the Anganwadi centres. A very large number of cases related to anemia are reported from all the AWCs in all the districts. Women between the ages 15 to 49 and babies between the ages of 6 to 36 months are found to be anemic in large number. The National Goitre Control programme is in operation in only Srikakulam, Vizianagaram and Mahboobnagar Districts with the other districts in the negative. In fact a very large number of Goitre cases were reported from Visakhapatnam District two/three decades ago due to iodine deficiency. Iodized salt supply was reported in all the PHCs of all the districts except in West Godavari and Khammam. A few Vitamin A deficiency disorders were reported especially for bitot spots and softening of cornea.

Table 3.6: Nutrition Disorders Reported from AWC

S. No.	District	How many in the Age Group of 6-35 months are Anaemic	15-49 Years Women are Anaemic	NGCP Operated		Goitre Cases	Iodized Salt Supply		Vitamin A Deficiency Disorder	
				Y	N		Y	N	A	B
1.	SR	532	976	4	—	3	—	4	6	3
2.	VM	104	152	4	--	4	—	4	—	4
3.	VS	120	80	—	11	2	—	11	—	—
4.	EG	12	131	—	14	8	10	4	—	—
5.	WG	147	127	—	6	—	6	—	—	—
6.	KA	50	532	—	5	—	5	—	—	—
7.	NE	186	296	—	3	—	2	1	—	12
8.	MN	—	—	1	1	—	—	2	—	—
9.	CU	144	310	—	2	5	—	2	—	—

SK: *Srikakulam;* VZ: *Vizianagaram;* VS: *Visakhapatnam;* EG: *East Godavari;* WG: *West Godavari;* KA: *Khammam;* NL: *Nellore;* MN: *Mahaboobnagar;* CU: *Cuddapah;* A: *softening of cornea;* B: *bitot spots are reported; AWC: Angan Wadi Centres;* NGCP: *National Goitre Control Programme.*

From Table 3.6.1 the performance of Anganwadi centres could be seen. In all the AWCs nutritious supplements such as dal, oil and rice are being provided. In addition services like periodic health check ups, immunizations, growth promoting supplementary feeding, referral services, early childhood care and pre-school education and distribution of nutrition supplements to promote child health are being provided. Only in a few place periodic health check-ups and immunizations are not regularly done as found in the AWCs of Cuddapah, Visakhapatnam and Mahboobnagar districts. It may be noted here that apart from the distribution of nutrition supplements, the AWC is the hub for the delivery of primary health care interventions by the ANM such as immunization, distribution of Iron and Folic Acid and Vitamin A supplements, distribution of oral contraceptive pills, growth monitoring and promotion and health education and counselling to mothers.

Table 3.7 presents data related to different health programmes initiated and implemented by the Government of India. It can be seen from Table 3.7 that the National Nutritional Anaemia

Table 3.6.1: Performance of Anganwadi Centres

S. No.	District	Nutrition Supplements provided			AWC these Services provided for Children						Functions of AWC		Describe the Mid Day Meal Programme		Do the AWC serve as Immunization and Supplementary Feed for 6 Months to 2 years	
		A	B	C	D	E	F	G	H	I	Y	N	Y	N	Y	N
1.	SR	4	4	4	4	4	4	4	4	4	4	—	4	—	4	—
2.	VM	4	4	4	2	2	4	2	4	4	4	—	4	—	4	—
3.	VS	11	11	7	—	5	7	4	10	—	6	5	8	3	7	4
4.	EG	14	14	14	3	6	14	5	14	2	9	5	10	4	11	3
5.	WG	6	6	6	2	6	6	6	6	6	6	—	6	—	6	—
6.	KA	5	5	5	5	5	2	4	3	5	5	—	5	—	5	—
7.	NE	3	3	3	3	3	3	3	3	3	3	—	3	—	3	—
8.	MN	2	2	2	—	—	2	2	2	2	1	1	1	1	1	1
9.	CU	2	2	2	—	—	2	2	2	2	1	1	1	1	1	1

SK: *Srikakulam;* VZ: *Vizianagaram;* VS: *Visakhapatnam;* EG: *East Godavari;* WG: *West Godavari;* KA: *Khammam;* NL: *Nellore;* MN: *Mahaboobnagar;* CU: *Cuddapah;* A: *rice* ; B: *dal;* C: *oil;* D: *health checkups;* E: *immunization;* F: *growth promotion and supplementary feeding;* G: *referral services;* H: *early childhood care and pre-school education;* I: *nutrition and child health.*

Prophylaxis Programme (NNAP) is in operation in all the PHCs in all the districts in our study except in 7 PHCs of Visakhapatnam District and 9 in East Godavari District. It can also be seen from Table 3.7 that in all the PHCs studied IFA (Iron and Folic Acid) tablets are being distributed to the pregnant women. The blindness prevention programme is in operation in all the PHCs except in 9 PHCs in Visakhapatnam District. Table 3.7 also speaks of the role of ASHA in the distribution of tablets for common illnesses like cough, cold and fever, rendering assistance to the ANMS, and imparting health education to the villagers, etc. According to the table a large number of TB cases were reported from Vizianagaram and Srikakulam Districts and the causative factors are found to be the

Table 3.7: Different Health Programmes

District	NNAP Operated		IFA Supplied		Prevention of Blindness Programme is operated		Role of ASHA			Prevalence of TB		
	Y	N	Y	N	Y	N	A	B	C	D	E	F
SR	4	—	4	—	4	—	4	4	4	4	4	95ca
VM	4	—	4	—	4	—	4	4	4	4	4	200
VS	4	7	11	—	2	9	11	11	—	11	6	4
EG	5	9	14	—	14	—	14	14	8	14	10	6
WG	6	—	6	—	6	—	6	6	4	6	6	—
KA	5	—	5	—	5	—	5	5	5	—	—	—
NE	3	—	3	—	3	—	3	3	3	—	—	—
MN	2	—	2	—	2	—	2	2	2	—	—	—
CU	2	—	2	—	2	—	2	2	2	—	—	—

SK: *Srikakulam*; VZ: *Vizianagaram*; VS: *Visakhapatnam*; EG: *East Godavari*; WG: *West Godavari*; KA: *Khammam*; NL: *Nellore;* MN: *Mahaboobnagar*; CU: *Cuddapah*; A: *tablets distribution*; B: *assistance of ANM*; C: *health education*; D: *smoking*; E: *food;* F: *conjucted rooms*.

habit of smoking, the types of foods they consume and living in crowded and congested rooms.

Table 3.8 gives the incidence of diarrhoea and other vector borne diseases which are locally endemic and the measures taken are such as the spraying of DDT, etc. As malaria is endemic all over India, the National Malaria Control Programme (NMCP) emphasizes the indoor residual spraying of DDT. It can be seen from Table 3.8 that all the PHCs in all the districts have reported the use of DDT spraying in their jurisdiction. It may be noted here that the prevalence of malaria is very high among the tribal communities and the Malarial experiences of the tribals is dealt with separately.

The diarrhoeal episodes are very common among the tribals and the etiology could be traced to consumption of contaminated water. The water shortages in many of the areas compound the situation further. In our study, the highest number of such cases was reported from Visakhapatnam, East Godavari, West Godavari and Nellore in that order. DOTS coverage refers to the number of cases covered under DOTS (Directly Observed Treatment-Short Course) under the revised National Tuberculosis Control Programme (RNTCP). East Godavari, Khammam, Nellore,

Table 3.8: Prevention and Control of Locally Endemic Diseases

District	DOTS Coverage Area	Diarrhoeal Episodes per year	Incidence of Vector Borne Diseases						DDT Spraying	
			A	B	C	D	E	F	Y	N
SR	4	1 time	270	3	-	-	4	-	4	-
VM	200	1	192	1	-	-	-	94	4	-
VS	64	3658	2581	5	-	-	-	10	11	-
EG	298	864	2383	-	-	-	-	30	14	-
WG	103	650	501	6	-	-	-	16	6	-
KA	245	32	-	-	-	-	-	11	5	-
NE	220	340	519	-	-	-	-	7	3	-
MN	40	1	-	-	-	-	-	3	2	-
CU	40	138	36	-	-	-	-	13	2	-

SK: *Srikakulam;* VZ: *Vizianagaram;* VS: *Visakhapatnam;* EG: *East Godavari;* WG: *West Godavari;* KA: *Khammam;* NL: *Nellore;* MN: *Mahaboobnagar;* CU: *Cuddapah;* A: *malaria;* B: *radesh;* C: *radesh encephalitis;* D: *Dengue;* E: *chickungunya;* F: *leprosy*

Vizianagaram and West Godavari reported highest coverage under DOTS. A very high number of vector borne diseases was reported from Visakhapatnam and East Godavari Districts.

Table 3.8.1 gives an account of the diarrhoeal deaths reported from the PHCs studied. It can be seen from the table that a few such cases were reported from Visakhapatnam (4), East Godavari (6), and West Godavari (2). In all the PHCs administration of ORS solution to prevent dehydration was reported.

One of the essential components of the Primary Health Care approach is the appropriate treatment of common illnesses and injuries at the peripheral level. An ANM manning the sub-centre is provided with prophylactic Kit A and essential drugs Kit B to manage such common illnesses. ARIs (acute respiratory infections) and diarrhoea are the two leading causes of childhood morbidity and mortality. Kit A contains IFA (large and small), Vitamin A solution, cotrimoxazole tablets, ORS packets, disposable delivery kit; Kit B contains methyl ergometrine maleate tablets/injection, paracetamol tablets, mebendazole, dicyclomine tablets, chloamphenicol eye ointment, povidone Iodine, cetrimide powder, cotton and bandages. All the ANMs in the study area have reported to carry these kits in all the PHCs in all the districts.

Table 3.8.1: PHC Staff, Diarrhoea Episodes etc.

District	ANMs carrying Kit A and Kit B		PHC Staff trained to Diagnose		Diarrhoea Deaths	ORS Solution administered	
	Y	N	Y	N		Y	N
SR	4	—	4	—	—	4	—
VM	4	—	4	—	—	4	—
VS	11	—	2	9	4	11	—
EG	14	—	9	5	6	14	—
WG	6	—	6	—	2	6	—
KA	5	—	5	—	—	5	—
NE	3	—	3	—	—	3	—
MN	2	—	2	—	—	2	—
CU	2	—	2	—	—	2	—

SK: *Srikakulam*; VZ: *Vizianagaram*; VS: *Visakhapatnam*; EG: *East Godavari*; WG: *West Godavari*; KA: *Khammam*; NL: *Nellore*; MN: *Mahaboobnagar;* CU: *Cuddapah.*

Table 3.9 gives data related to the treatment of common diseases and injuries. All the PHCs reported that ORS packets are available with them. The ORS meant for mothers also is available in all the PHCs except 2 in Visakhapatnam, 3 in East Godavari and 1 in West Godavari. In addition to ORS, Zinc tablets are also supplied except in 2 PHCs in Visakhapatnam and 6 in East Godavari District. ASHA is found to be active in all the villages under the PHCs studied except in Visakhapatnam and East Godavari Districts. Kit A and Kit B details are already dealt with and in all the PHCs the kits contain the medications as described in Table 3.9.

Table 3.9.1 gives additional information related to treatment of common illnesses and injuries. IMNCI refers to Integrated Management of Neo-natal and Childhood illnesses and all the PHCs studied reported that there have been following IMNCI except in case of 11 PHCs in Visakhapatnam and 5 in East Godavari District. The syndromic based diagnosis is practiced by all the health workers in all the PHCs except in Visakhapatnam and a few in East Godavari (4) and West Godavari (3). Kits for sexually Transmitted Infections (STI) are in good supply in all the PHCs except in Srikakulam District. All the PHCs have reported that the drugs are available on a regular basis in their centres. The list of essential drugs is incomplete with only PHCs in Srikakulam

Table 3.9: Treatment of Common Illness and Injuries

District	*Mother Oriented ORS Solution*		*ORS available with Health Workers*		*Supply Zinc Tablets as an Adjunct to ORS*		*ASHA deal with Generic Ailments*		*Following provided with the Drug Kit to deliver First Contact Health Care*										
	Y	N	Y	N	Y	N	Y	N	A	B	C	D	E	F	G	H	I	J	K
SR	4	—	4	—	4	—	4	—	4	4	4	4	4	4	4	4	4	4	4
VM	4	—	4	—	4	—	4	—	4	4	4	4	4	4	4	4	4	4	4
VIZ	9	2	11	—	9	2	—	11	11	11	11	11	11	11	11	11	11	11	11
EG	11	3	14	—	8	6	—	14	14	14	14	14	14	14	14	14	14	14	14
WG	5	1	6	—	6	—	4	2	6	6	6	6	6	6	6	6	6	6	6
KA	5	—	5	—	5	—	5	—	5	5	5	5	5	5	5	5	5	5	5
NE	3	—	3	—	3	—	3	—	3	3	3	3	3	3	3	3	3	3	3
MN	2	—	2	—	2	—	2	—	—	2	2	2	2	2	2	2	2	2	2
CU	2	—	2	—	2	—	2	—	2	2	2	2	2	2	2	2	2	2	2

SK: *Srikakulam;* VZ: *Vizianagaram;* VS: *Visakhapatnam;* EG: *East Godavari;* WG: *West Godavari;* KA: *Khammam;* NL: *Nellore;* MN: *Mahaboobnagar;* CU: *Cuddapah;* A: *kit A-IFA (large and small), vitamin A solution;* B: *cotrimoxazole tablets;* C: *ORS packets;* D: *disposable delivery kit;* E: *2 kit B; F-methyl ergometrine maleate tablets/injection;* G: *paracetamol tablets, tab. Mebendazole, tab dicyclomine;* H: *amphenicoleye ointment;* I: *ointment povidone iodine;* J: *cetrimide powder;* K: *cotton and bandages provided with a drug kit.*

District providing information which reflects on the ignorance of in PHC staff as to what we mean by 'essential drugs'. In fact the kits A and B contain most of the essential drugs.

Table 3.10 refers to the supply of kits and the availability of standard treatment guidelines in the PHCs. Table 3.10 also gives information related to their staff having got in-service training. It can be seen from the table that all the Sub-Centers of the PHCs of this study are being supplied with the kits containing essential drugs every six months. The availability of standard treatment guidelines was answered in the positive by all the PHCs except 1 in Srikakulam District, 2 in Vizianagaram and 4 in Visakhapatnam PHCs. With regard to the in-service training of the PHC staff except in case of 7 PHCs in Visakhapatnam, 8 in East Godavari, 2 in West Godavari Districts, all other PHCs reported in the positive.

Table 3.9.1: Treatment of Common Illness and Injuries

District	IMNCI followed		Health Worker Practice Syndromic Based Diagnosis		Supply STI Kits		List of Essential Drugs		Drugs are available on Regular Basis	
	Y	N	Y	N	Y	N	Y	N	Y	N
SR	4	—	3	1	—	4	4	—	4	—
VM	4	—	3	—	2	—	—	—	4	—
VS	—	11	—	11	11	—	—	—	11	—
EG	9	5	10	4	14	—	—	—	14	—
WG	6	—	3	3	6	—	—	—	6	—
KA	5	—	5	—	5	—	—	—	5	—
NE	3	—	3	—	3	—	—	—	3	—
MN	2	—	2	—	2	—	—	—	2	—
CU	2	—	2	—	2	—	—	—	2	—

SK: *Srikakulam*; VZ: *Vizianagaram*; VS: *Visakhapatnam*; EG: *East Godavari*; WG: *West Godavari*; KA: *Khammam*; NL: *Nellore*; MN: *Mahaboobnagar*; CU: *Cuddapah*.

Table 3.10: Provision of Essential Drugs

District	Sub-Centres Supply Kits Every Six Months		Strategies Adopted for Safe and Rational Use of Drugs		PHC Staff got any in-service Training		You got Standard Treatment Guidelines	
	Y	N	Y	N	Y	N	Y	N
SR	4	—	—	—	4	—	3	1
VM	4	—	—	—	4	—	2	2
VS	11	—	—	—	4	7	7	4
EG	14	—	—	—	6	8	14	—
WG	6	—	—	—	4	2	6	—
KA	5	—	—	—	5	—	5	—
NE	3	—	—	—	3	—	3	—
MN	2	—	—	—	2	—	2	—
CU	2	—	—	—	2	—	2	—

SK: *Srikakulam*; VZ: *Vizianagaram*; VS: *Visakhapatnam*; EG: *East Godavari*; WG: *West Godavari*; KA: *Khammam*; NL: *Nellore*; MN: *Mahaboobnagar*; CU: *Cuddapah*.

Table 3.11 refers to the water supply and sanitation in the villages within the jurisdiction of the PHCs in this study. From Table 3.11 it can be seen that the paramedical staff of the PHCs are attending to the problems related to the sanitation within the villages with the exception of 2 PHCs in Vizianagaram District. However it may be noted here in all the villages defecation is done in the open places as access to toilets is almost negligible in the study villages. It can also be seen from that table that they are in the practice of imparting health education to the villagers with the exception of 5 PHCs in Visakhapatnam District. When the question of their awareness of the essential drugs devised by Indian Public Health standards they all have invariably replied in the positive. With reference to their knowledge related to the protocols for diarrhoea and immunization schedules they all have replied in the positive. It is only in case of TB, 8 PHCs and in case of leprosy 11 PHCs all in Visakhapatnam replied in the negative.

Table 3.11: Water Supply and Sanitation

District	*Para medical Staff Address the Question of Sanitation in the Village*		*They Impart Any Health Education to the Tribals*		*Aware of the Essential Drugs devised by Indian Public Health Standard*		*Know the Protocol for the following*							
	Y	*N*	*Y*	*N*	*Y*	*N*	*A*		*B*		*C*		*D*	
SR	4	—	4	—	4	—	4	—	4	—	4	—	4	—
VM	2	2	4	—	4	—	4	—	4	—	4	—	4	—
VS	11	—	6	5	11	—	3	8	11	—	—	11	11	—
EG	14	—	14	—	14	—	14	—	14	—	14	—	14	—
WG	6	—	6	—	6	—	6	—	6	—	6	—	6	—
KA	5	—	5	—	5	—	5	—	5	—	5	—	5	—
NE	3	—	3	—	3	—	3	—	3	—	3	—	3	—
MN	2	—	2	—	2	—	2	—	2	—	2	—	2	—
CU	2	—	2	—	2	—	2	—	2	—	2	—	2	—

SK: *Srikakulam;* VZ: *Vizianagaram;* VS: *Visakhapatnam;* EG: *East Godavari;* WG: *West Godavari;* KA: *Khammam;* NL: *Nellore;* MN: *Mahaboobnagar;* CU: *Cuddapah;* A: *TB;* B: *diarrhoea;* C: *leprosy;* D: *other immunization schedules.*

Table 3.12 refers to the activities of the PHCs in imparting health education to their patients as well as the villagers under their jurisdiction. All the staff of the PHCs in one voice have replied that they are engaged in the activities related to the prevention of HIV/AIDs and other life-style diseases. The IEC (Information, education and communication) activities included pasting wall posters and catchy slogans wherever possible in addition to arranging rallies periodically to create more and more awareness about these diseases. Monitoring of the impact of these activities is also undertaken by all the PHCs. Health melas are organized periodically in all the PHCs invariably.

Table 3.12: Health Education

District	*Engage in Preventing HIV and Other Life Style Diseases*		*List of IEC Interventions*			*Contextual Needs*		*Any Training Health Workers In Inter Personal Communication*		*Monitor Impact of IEC*		*Health Melas organised*		*Inherent Drawbacks*	
	Y	*N*	*A*	*B*	*C*	*D*	*E*	*Y*	*N*	*Y*	*N*	*Y*	*N*	*Y*	*N*
SR	4	—	4	4	4	4	4	4	—	4	—	4	—	4	—
VM	4	—	4	4	4	4	—	4	—	4	—	4	—	4	—
VS	11	—	11	11	—	11	—	—	11	11	—	11	—	11	—
EG	14	—	14	14	8	14	—	7	7	14	—	14	—	14	—
WG	6	—	6	6	6	6	6	6	6	6	—	6	—	3	3
KA	5	—	5	5	5	—	—	5	—	5	—	5	—	5	—
NE	3	—	3	3	3	—	—	2	—	3	—	3	—	3	—
MN	2	—	2	2	2	—	—	2	—	2	—	2	—	2	—
CU	2	—	2	2	2	—	—	2	—	2	—	2	—	2	—

SK: *Srikakulam*; VZ: *Vizianagaram*; VS: *Visakhapatnam*; EG: *East Godavari*; WG: *West Godavari*; KA: *Khammam*; NL: *Nellore*; MN: *Mahaboobnagar*; CU: *Cuddapah*; A: *wall posters*; B: *slogans*; C: *rallies*; D: *staff*; E: *medicine budget*.

Gender Differences

It is observed many a time during the fieldwork in tribal villages that in general there is a preference for male child to a girl child. This is reflected in the treatment meted out to them especially in feeding practices. The boys and men are fed first and then only the girls and the women. This tendency was found mostly among the Savaras, Gadabas, Porjas and Kondhs, all primitive tribes. The more a tribe is primitive the more is such a tendency. The Valmikis and the Bagathas are at the other end of the spectrum and found to be more advanced among the tribal communities of Andhra Pradesh.

IV

The Tribal Medicine Man (The Shaman)

Systematic studies conducted on the tribes of Eastern Ghats demonstrate distinct cultural differences among these tribes. Although cultural differences abound some similarities in the area of religion are not uncommon. Tribal religion in these parts of India is mostly animistic although the influence of Hinduism is seen in some religious practices. Invoking divine beings for blessings is a common practice at the time of agricultural operations, i.e., sowing and harvesting. In the area of Health too dependence on divinatory forces is distinctly visible in their curative practices. The tribals believe that different elements, conditions, and persons are responsible for different types of ailments such as the natural causes, breach of taboo and social regulations, ancestral spirits, sorcerers and witches, malevolent spirits etc. For example, the Savaras and Jatapus strong belief in these supernaturai beings is expressed in the representations drawn on the walls or on the ground sometimes erecting a platform or altar near the house to drive away the evil spirits.

Hemant Bag and Kapoor (2007: 37-48) reported the magico-religious practices among the Kondhs in the treatment of diseases: It was reported that 20.71 per cent of Kondhs first approach their tribal practitioner who is locally called Guru/Gunia, Pujari for their treatment. The Gunia or Guru represents a particular deity. When the deity appears through him, his body starts shivering rapidly and his contact with this world breaks for a short span of time. During such moments he speaks out the causes of ailments and suggests remedies. He performs the following rites in succession :

1. First throws some raw rice over the patient after reciting some spells, then he gives spiritual ash (*char*) purified by reciting *mantras* (incantations).
2. If he is not cured then a thread is tied around his arms.
3. If this does not produce any result then chicken or pigeon are sacrificed.
4. If still it does not help, goat or lamb sacrifice is performed.
5. If a patient does not get cured, then he/she is taken to the PHC.

For the epidemic diseases like cholera and small pox they also perform ritual at the community level. On the appointed day, all the villagers are assembled in the *'Dhurni'* the worship place. Each family offers *mudhi* and ghee and fire. On behalf of the villagers one chicken and pigeon are sacrificed.

Behura and Mohanty (2006: 100-143) report classification of human diseases among the Koya and Saora of Orissa on the basis of symptoms. The Koya magico-religious and ethno-medicinal specialist is designated as Wadde, who diagnoses and treats diseases is usually a man, but could be a woman also. There is a hierarchical gradation among them: the junior shaman or shamanin is known as *Roto wadde,* the intermediate specialists are called *Sira wadde,* and the senior ones are designated as *Berry wadde.* Whereas among the Saora, Shamanins, called Kudanboi, are numerically preponderant. There are both magico-religious experts and medicine specialist, who are only men and are designated as *reogammar*.

The indigenous system of diagnosis among the Koya is called *pentasyad* and among Saora it is called *tedum*. Koyas have an elaborate system of classification of diseases, such as, (i) child diseases or *sodupillarooum,* (ii) male diseases or *nurrogum,* (iii) female diseases or *detarooum,* (iv) old age diseases or *musulwadrogum,* (v) mental diseases or *verrooum,* (vi) dental diseases or *andarooum,* (vii) nail diseases or *reybubarooum,* (viii) ear diseases or *ashudahurooum,* (ix) eye diseases or *iamatrooum,* (x) seasonal diseases or *Kaalamrooum,* and (xi) skin diseases or *talkarogum*. Saoras do not classify diseases. And neither Saora nor Koya classify diseases as contagious, infectious, air borne or water borne. But they have some notion of hereditary diseases as well as incurable diseases.

Mohanty and Mahapatra (2005: 1-11) report that the very word Saora owe to *Sagories*, a radesh word meaning axe and *Saba-Roye*, a Sanskrit word meaning carrying a dead body (hunted animal) links the tribe with hunting and collecting activities in the distant past. Like any other tribe the Saora measure health or illness of a person in terms of food intake and work output. The traditional Saora medical provider is known as *Kudan* or *Kudanboi*. The former is a male shaman while the latter is the female counterpart. Every Saora village has a *Kudan* or *Kudanboi* and the patient need not go outside the village for treatment.

The Dongria Kondh is a primitive and backward section of the Kondh tribe. Their age old institution of Shamanism still has a powerful influence on them and their male and female shamans are called *Beju* and *Bejuni* (*Pejuni*) respectively. They are the most distinguished and respected magico-religious functionaries in their society (Gamango, 2007: 139-149).

Jhansi Rani (2009) documents that the medicine men in most cases among the Bondo are males. Good medicine men, for his ability to heal the ailing persons, attain the status of a folk hero. A Bondo woman may serve medicine—both material and institutional—but she is seldom addressed as a *Gurumai* or *Dissari*. During pre- and post-marriage period a female may learn the symptoms of the disease and prepare antidotes (medicine).

In the Bondo country the medicine men are classified into three broad groups namely the *Guru*, the *Dissari* and those laymen who have mastered the use of certain plants, animals and minerals. No specific name has been given to the medicine man of latter category. In a *guru* one finds the heredity of both the medicine manship. A *Dissari* is an astrologer-*cum*-medicineman who prescribes indigenous medicines and performs magical rituals. He has a good knowledge about the causes of diseases and the treatments. The *Dissari* usually takes care of seasonal and endemic diseases and body disorders caused by visible agents. When a person faces accidents repeatedly or in cyclic order the *Dissari* applies some herbal medicines but to boost the moral of the patient he performs some rituals too. These rituals may not have any clinical effect but boost confidence and build up the will to survive.

Interpretation of illness is a culturally informed process, one in which patient, healer and a community of others make use of locally appropriate disease theories to account for the misfortune at hand. Disease theories in non-western societies may emphasize naturalistic origins or they may attribute misfortune to the workings of a "personalistic" agent like a god, an ancestral ghost, or a vengeful human (Foster, 1976). That personalistic, naturalistic etiological systems are not mutually exclusive is recognized in many studies abroad and also among tribals in India (Saurez, 1974; Hymavathi, 1996; Nanda Kishore, 1999; Karteek, 1992). The disease etiologies in tribal societies often typically make a distinction between immediate and ultimate clause. The former provides details on the specific nature of the problem and the latter offers a rationalization as to why this problem occurred. Referring to Goody's observations based on the study among la Dagaa of Ghana (Goody, 1962), Foster describes how personalistic systems are more complex in that two or more levels of causality can be distinguished and in curing, these levels must be taken into account. Disease etiologies, of course, reflect the world views of the members of a society and also correlate with the nature of economic and political organization of societies (Snow, 1974; Foster, 1976: 454).

Savara Conception of Health, Disease and Etiology of Disease

They attribute any misfortune, including disease and death, to the displeasure of their supreme supernatural being *Jamaraju*, or of other lesser gods or of their ancestors. It is widely believed among them that supernatural beings cause disease as a punishment for any immoral behaviour or violation of social norms (Madhav Krishna, 1995).

Obeyesekere (1969) opines that the Savara disease etiology offers a dual taxonomy for an identical disease, in one it may be due to supernatural or human agent and in another or for the same person at a later time, simply a natural agent. As beliefs of supernatural causation of disease and also belief in sorcery and witchcraft resulting in illness prevail very much, the magico-religious healers will have a significant role to play in the Savara society.

The Savaras and Jatapus of Srikakulam District believe in four types of spirits: (1) Protective Spirits or deities such as *Ammathalli*, Goddalamma or goddess of axe, and Kuchalamma, etc., (2) Benevolent spirits such as Loddalu, Kondathalli *loddalu, Desi loddalu, Inti* (house) *loddalu, Panta* (crop) *loddalu, Kotem* (non-local) *loddalu,* who are worshipped by every family to safeguard themselves from disease, death and other calamities; (3) Malevolent spirits like *Ammavaru, Ganyo, Gusada, Sathalamma* (*Thokkidi Devatha*), *Kannibojan-Jammaraju, Kanni,* etc, who control smallpox, fever, abortions etc; (4) All the ancestral spirits such as, *Bhootha, Peeri, Pisachi,* etc., who are benevolent in protecting the family members.

The medicine man is locally called as *Yejjodu*/Yejjuralu in Srikakulam District (Rajpramukh, 1976) and *Guru* or *Goragadu,* etc., in Visakhapatnam District. The medicine man is a part time magico-religious specialist adept at trans-divination, curing by magical power directly from a supernatural source. An important element of the shaman's work is the performance of public (rather private) rituals, in which divination and curing are accomplished through trance. When sickness is not cured for many days the patients approach the shaman for cure, who is familiar with local medicinal herbs, trees, barks, and pastes made out of crushed leaves. Warding of devils and demons is their speciality and a typical tribal believes in the existence of these spirits and spirit possession of individuals. They also believe in black magic and the first bout of sickness is suspected to be the handiwork of a shaman.

Many tribals in Munchingput mandal wear a charm around their neck. It immediately indicates that such a person was suffering from some disease and that he was being treated by the shaman. Almost every other kid in tribal villages wears this charm around their neck which shows their profound faith in the healing power of the shaman. The fees usually collected by the shaman include a bottle or two of native liquor, a hen besides a small fees, which varies from Rs. 10 to Rs. 300 depending upon the financial position of the patient.This practice of patronizing the shaman still continues despite the fact that the government opened many primary health centres (P.H.C's) with qualified medical doctors at many places in the tribal areas. It is mostly because of the fear in the tribal mind of the shaman's powers to deal with the evil spirits and engage these to fulfil any of their purposes. The medical officer in the P.H.C. at Muchingput confirmed that many patients are brought into the P.H.C. at a critical stage of the disease; their first approach invariably is to the local shaman. The shaman thus wields enormous influence in the lives of tribals in dealing with sickness.

While the belief system influences the perception of disease and accordingly bring in the shaman as much preferred over the modern medicine man, some behavioural practices also contributes to the outbreak of diseases. For example, in Jodiput, inhabited by Malis, the tribals have a practice of defecating in the open on the hill top at the bottom of which their villages is located. It is reported by the PHC medical doctor that in this village there is an unusual rate of the incidence of water borne diseases like, gastro-enteritis, amoebiasis, bacillary dysentery and occasionally cholera. It seems during the rainy seasons, the water that flows down the hill carrying the human faeces is collected in the tank at the bottom of the hill near the village and the same water is being used by tribals for drinking purpose which is the etiological factor for the abnormal rate of water borne diseases among them.

It is also found that sexual behaviour also plays a vital role in the etiology and transmission of diseases. Among many of the tribals, there is a high prevalence of pre-marital and extra-marital relationships. For example among the Porjas of Shrujanapeta, it is reported that young boys of about 13-14 years old indulge in sexual relations even with girls older than their age. It is also reported in some cases that younger boys of 8 or 9 years old also have their own girl friends. In yet another instance, while the sons are still in their tender years, the fathers marry girls on behalf of their sons. While it is beyond the scope of this study to deal in detail with the marital practices and sexual relations prevalent among these tribals, it becomes necessary here to touch upon some salient features of their sexual life as they pose health problems of unmanageable proportion. It is reported, as the average Porja is drawn into sexual life at an early age and is constantly engaged in it, by the time they reach 30 or 35 years age, they all become 'old'and eventually die at a relatively younger age.

The loose sexual code of conduct among some of the tribals is taken advantage of by the outsiders. For instance, after a battalion of Reserve Police were posted in Munchingput to contain the Naxalite problem in 1990, there was a rapid increase in the sexually transmitted diseases reported at the Munchingput PHC. Problems of this kind could be easily controlled if necessary precautions are taken in checking the contact between tribals and others.

For them the spirits are of two kinds: there are malevolent spirits as well as benevolent spirits. Spirits become malevolent, when they were not appeased properly or by performing the death ceremony. It could be due to negligence in the performance of the death ceremony or due to defective performance of the ceremony. The malevolent spirits are not propitiated but are feared with repulsion. They try to counter and tame them with the help of the shaman.

Table 4.1: The Supernatural Beings of Eastern Ghats Tribals associated with Diseases

Name of Supernatural being	*Diseases Associated*
Korangi Gurdi	Chills and fevers; diseases that originate from the hills and gales
Bhima Gurdi	Bites of poisonous lizards and insects
Gangamma Debta	Measles; general welfare
Jhanker Debta	Diseases of the forest; ill-health due to eating poisonous leaves, fruits and nuts
Gorob Nisani	Fevers, weakness affecting resistance due to Jal kamni
Peda Ammavaru & Chinna Ammavaru	Smallpox; Chickenpox
Kannibhojan	Psychic disorders
Gusada	Vomitings

The evil spirits are called by different names (a long list): *Bhoota, Graha peeda, Shanipeeda, Vanukulapeeda, Maavelli, Telia Maavelli, Kondapeeda, Geddapeeda, Balagraham, Chandapeeda, Dumbapeeda, Chinugula Dumba, Konda dumba, Adavi peedalu, Sokudu peedalu, Puli bhootham, Chettu bhootham,* and *Kateru bhootham*. They believe that the evil spirits have the ability to appear in any form— in the form of a man or woman, with the feet pointing backwards and they look like a dazzling glow or a flame emitting sparks. "Besides the deities, it is also believed that the ancestral as well as the other spirits known as *Dumba* cause similar afflictions by casting their evil eye on the people. In Dongria community and other neighbouring communities a good number of *Dumbas* are known to cause harm. They are *Maradi Dumba, Mari Dumba, Danger Dumba, Danda Penka, Takranipenu,* and *Mahmi*. The favourite abodes of these evil spirits are believed to be trees, stones, old houses and hills. They can travel in air without being seen. Their most favourite haunting places are burial grounds and natural springs. They can be seen during nights and in twilight. The shaman of Visakhapatnam District believes that there is no hierarchy among these spirits. He asserts that he can confine and release the spirits by his magical spells.

The Shaman's Diagnostic Procedures and Techniques

According to the shaman in the North Coastal Andhra Agency areas of Eastern Ghats, whenever any person is possessed by these evil spirits, the person's pulse becomes very weak and his/her hands become cold as ice and the patient appears restless. The first step the shaman takes is to place a winnow containing burnt cow dung cake over the head of the patient. He inscribes the name of a popular god on this cow dung ash. Then invoking the name of his *Guru,* he chants some *mantras* to propitiate his spirit-familiar. Thus he commissions his spirit-familiar into the ash which now becomes sacred powder (*vibhoothi*) and smears it on the forehead of the patient. Then he takes a handful of this sacred powder and blows it over the head of his patient. Immediately the evil spirit leaves the patient and the patient regains full consciousness. If the spirit still refuses to leave the patient, the shaman mixes pepper powder with the juice extracted from *tulsi* leaves and smears it on the eyes of the patient. This medication causes burning sensation in the eyes and tears roll down the eyes of the patients relieving the spirit too. In this haunted condition the patient also would be able to reveal the name of the spirit when his little finger's nail is pressed hard.

If the sickness is due to sorcery or witchcraft, the shaman performs a prayer to invoke his spirit-familiar and decides the course of treatment. It is also believed that the spirits of the dead ancestors also appear in the dreams of either the patient or the shaman and are informed of the mode of treatment to be followed.

The shamans in this region also use *talismans*. They tie them around their neck or upper hand, even after warding off the evil spirits, to protect their patients from a relapse of ghost-haunting. The shamans also claim that they also protect houses from being haunted by evil spirits. Chanting of magical incantations is the first step they resort to, followed by fixing nine wooden nails in the nine corners of the house. His magical spell commissions the services of his spirit—familiar to drive away the ghost and the nine nails never allow the ghost to re-enter the house. The shaman, in order to be very effective, has to observe many taboos. He should not light his cigar with other man's lighted cigar. He should not participate in the communal feasts given during the death ceremonies. On Saturdays and Mondays, he is not supposed to eat meat. For his services he never demands any fees. Only voluntary offerings are accepted.

Before taking up the case to cure, the shaman conducts a test or *Akshintailu Choodadam* to know whether to take up the case or not. They take a handful of grains (any kind) and count them. If the number is even they know that they can cure the patient so the patient can be treated. But if the number is odd, they won't take up the case as they believe that the patient can't survive.

A rather interesting technique is followed to know whether the person is affected by black magic or not. They put some rice in a winnow (or a bowl) and look into the rice with sheer concentration. They say that, the image of the black magician, who is responsible for the patient's sickness, will appear to him, to him only, in the bowl.

To know whether the patient is affected by ghosts, spirits etc., they make the patient smell a dried herb *Adavi Pasupu*. If the patient feels no smell, it is believed that the patient was affected by a ghost. But if he feels a pungent and foul smell, he is considered normal and healthy. They, then use *Voocha Kommu* to throw away the evil spirit.

To know what kind of ghost or evil spirit is acting on a patient, they usually feel the pulse (*nadi*). Some specified parts in the palm have been given names. They hold the wrist of the patient with one hand, and study the points on the palm. At whatever point they feel the change, that point is the ghost, which is said to be responsible for the illness. Then they use the appropriate method to ward off that ghost.

To know the life chances of a person, bitten by a snake, they crush some kinds of leaves in their palms. If, it produces white foam, they believe that the patient would survive, but if only water comes without foam, the patient would, for sure, die. To detect leprosy, they rub the leaves of *Kodimala* on the suspected area of the body. If the patient feels itchy, the skin is normal, but if the patient feels no itching sensation, the skin is supposed to be infected with leprosy.

Treatment for Common Diseases

Many of the common diseases are treated with the locally available herbs; for example, for cold and cough, a powder made of *Devadar* bark, and locally called *Pherangi chekka* is used. The powder is mixed with water and is gulped. It is believed that this powder helps in better digestion too.

Similarly for whooping cough, the medicine man ties a Raksha (*Talisman*) around the neck of the child. This *Raksha* is in the form of a necklace, made out of the fibre of some local tree. If the cough is severe he gives *Tuniki Ginja.* These seeds have to be crushed into a fine powder and added with some water, made into a fine paste and administered into the child, orally. For measles, chicken pox, etc., the treatment is through the propitiation of local deities. The shaman performs a ritual and uses the flour of chollu, turmeric, and some kinds of flowers. During the ritual he chants *mantras* in front of the fire and throws *sambrani* (frankincense) into it. The smoke that emanates is diverted to the body of the patient and is believed to give relief. For epidemics, sacrificing of goats and chicken is practiced. In case of dog bites and other wounds, that particular bitten area is bound with a rope made of jute and some crushed herbs and medicinal leaves, placed and tied with a cloth.

When a person shows unusual symptoms and changes in behaviour and becomes weak gradually in spite of other curative measures, the people believe that he is affected with the *Dumba* (evil spirit). The medicine man possesses innate powers and based on the symptoms identified, a particular ancestor of a spirit is considered responsible for the ill health of the person. Then he follows a procedure to get into trance to identify the deceased ancestor. That procedure requires materials like *korra* flour, *sindhur,* turmeric powder, sambrani, eggs and different types of fruits and flowers. He also chants some *mantras.* The shaman is paid both in cash and articles. If the patient dies in spite of the shaman's efforts, the blame is passed on only to the powerful evil spirits, but not to the shaman.

The Designs the Shamans use to cure Patients

A very interesting feature among the tribes of Visakhapatnam District is that the shaman draws different designs for different illnesses, including warding off the spirits or ghosts. Some of the designs they draw for the treatment of different patients are given here:

For Kateru Ghost

It has 24 corners. This is to be drawn in the burial ground. with 3 colours red, black, white. At the centre, the head of a chicken is to be placed and also flowers, green peas, etc.

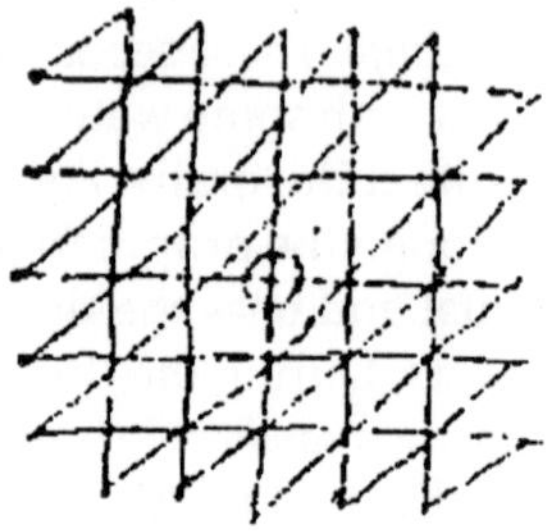

For Shani

This is to be drawn in *thatta* (basket). 3 pairs of white flowers, multi-coloured chick are required for this. The head of the chick is to be cut down and the blood sprinkled with the head in the design. The *thatta* is to be placed at cross roads before 7 AM.

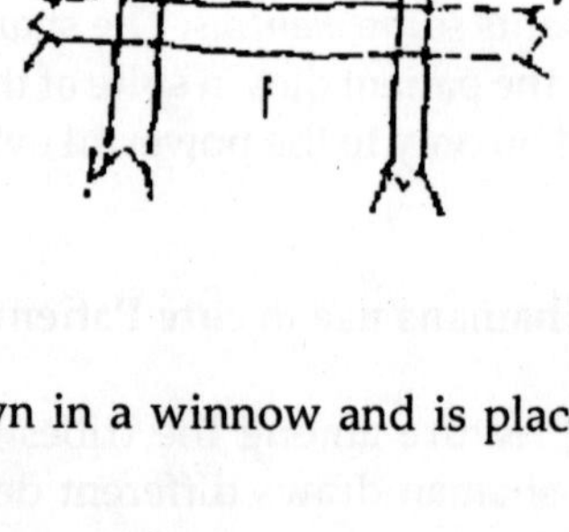

For Dishti Peeda

This is to be drawn in a winnow and is placed in the pathway commonly used.

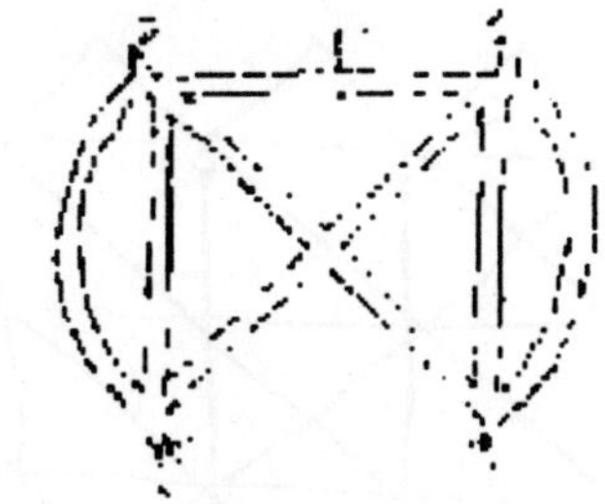

For Dishti Peeda

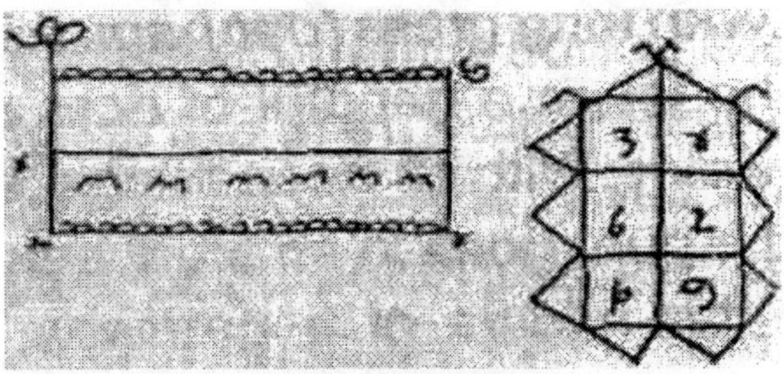

For Dhisti (Evil Eye)

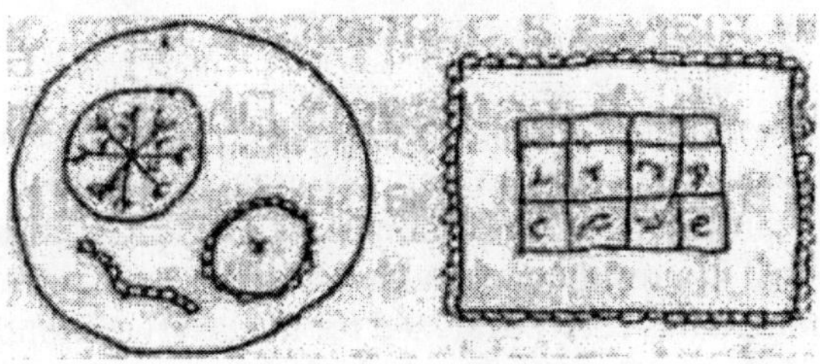

Toward off Ghosts

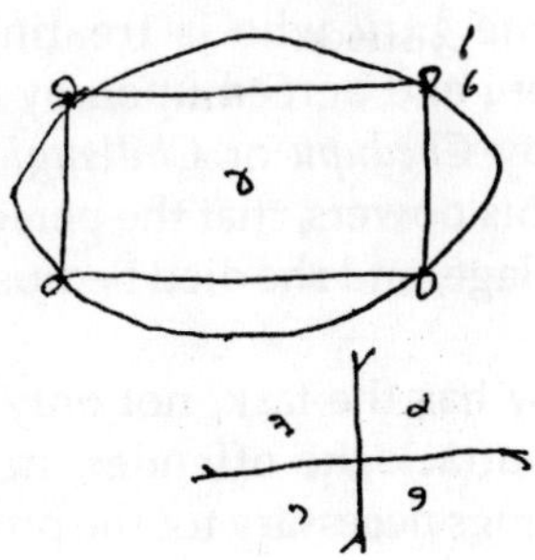

To drive away Shani (Jinx)

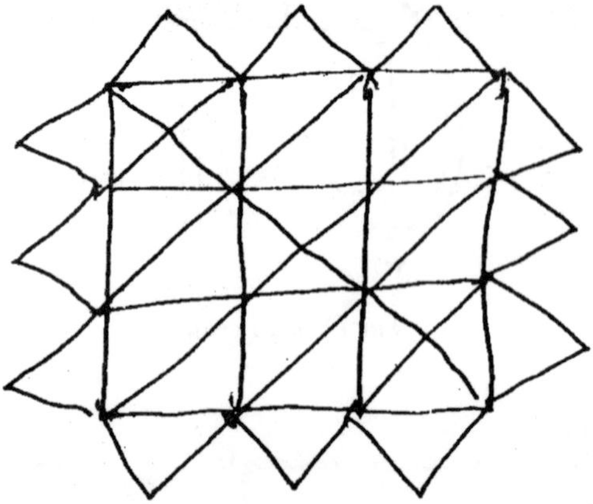

For Rahuvu (Bad Times)

Around the four corners of the design or *muggu*, they usually hang pieces of cloth. In the design or *muggu*, they (the shamans) usually use eggs, the head of a fowl, head of a dove, in case of Kondulu or Samantalu, but for Bagathas they use only flowers and chick.

Case Study

The patient is Kimudu Gonjibabu, aged 18 years. He is a resident of the village, Mettavalasa and belongs to Jatapu tribe. The medicine man's name is Surla Thomas, aged 50 years, also belongs to Jatapu and is a resident of Mettavalasa.

The patient has been paralyzed for the last two months on the left side. He can't sit erect even in bed. For everything he has to take the help from his parents. He was treated two times for other ailments by the same *guru* who is treating him now. It was diagnosed by the *guru* and agreed upon by the parents that the patient is affected by *Chedupu* or *Chillangi* (black magic). The shaman knew, with his powers, that the person who did this was a lady of a nearby village, and she died because of rivalry with the patient's family.

The shaman now has the task, not only to cure the patient but also to counter-attack the offender. In the collection and preparation of the things necessary for the procedure, the shaman is helped by the father and the mother of the patient. First of all, with bamboo like stems, the *Gummadi theega*, he makes a bow and three arrows. He then takes some red clay, to this he adds water, kneads the clay and then makes an idol of a female, which represents the woman who did the black magic to the patient. With long grass (*dabbagaddi*), he then makes a 5 stranded form or plait. Then he takes a handful of rice, a live crab, which represents *Dhakuni* and a potful of water. With all these things, along with the patient, the parents and his assistant, the *guru* goes to an area, selected carefully outside the village and exactly on the middle of a pathway. The assistant sprinkles water, lights scented sticks or *agarbathis* (incandescence) and by chanting *mantras* he makes some designs with red, black and/or white colours.

The shaman, then, draws two diagrams: 'a human being' and 'Bow and arrows'. An idol was placed on the diagram of human being, and on the other diagram real bow and arrows were placed. Afterwards he took a big leaf and on it drew the lines along its veins with red, black and white colours. Around the design he arranged 11 leaves and on the leaves he dropped small flowers of all colours. The leaves are Panduga, Karnada, Konda mamidi, Puruguda, and Parikika. Then he mixed the rice with red, white and black colours separately and placed the rice on the leaves. He also placed pieces of banana, some millets and cooked grains on the leaves. He lighted *pramida* (wick lamp) and kept it on the right side of the design. Then he made the patient sit on the design and then called loudly the gods and goddesses, he knew, to help. Cooked rice was thrown in all directions. The shaman then took out the crab and tied an oil rinsed cloth to its legs, lighted the cloth, and then kept the crab on the design. He took out a small chick and made it touch the patient's head, cut the beak of the chick, dropped blood from its beak on the design and finally cut the head of the chicken, kept it on the design and threw the remaining body away. He took out the 5 strand-grass and with it he brushed the patient's body from head to toe, while chanting *mantras* in Oriya. Then he cut the grass into pieces and threw them on the design. Then with a single strand of grass, he repeated the same process.

He took out a book malayala mantram in Telugu and from it chanted several *mantras* for a long time. After that he tied oiled cloth to arrows, lighted them and shot them, two over the patient's head and one over his own head. Then he cut the nose of the idol. Afterwards, he mixed a drug made from several herbs, with water and made the patient to drink it. Later, he took a green branch, spat on it and put it on the pathway. Then he sent the patient home, collected all his belongings and the chick's head and body. Later he announced that the patient is going to be cured within three days and the woman who is responsible for the black magic is going to suffer the same as the patient.

V

Health Care Delivery System and Tribals' Diseases

Health care system for the tribals in Andhra Pradesh follows the same system that is meant for all other populations. The three basic operational components are the sub-centres (SC), primary health centres (PHCs), and the first referral units, i.e., the community health centres (CHCs). The district medical and health officer (DM and HO) is responsible for all matters related to administration and programme management at district level. He functions under the control of Commissioner, Family Welfare, Government of Andhra Pradesh.

Visakhapatnam District is divided into three divisions for administrative convenience, viz., Visakhapatnam, Narsipatnam and Paderu. Among these three the Paderu division covers the agency or tribal area of the district. There are at present 32 PHCs in the Paderu division catering to the health needs of the tribal population. In addition to these there are three CHCs, one in Paderu and the other two in Araku and Chintapalli.

A few of the PHCs all over the State are converted into 24 hours maternity health care centres where the services of a gynaecologist and a paediatrician are available and such health centers provide maternity and child care services round the clock. A sample of the action taken by the D.H.M.O. in East Godavari District for the year 2007-2008 is presented here:

1. First Round General spray completed from 15.04.2007 to 31-5-2007 covered 461 villages out of 669 villages with a population of 1,42,579.

2. Second Round General spray completed from 01.06.2007 to 25.8.2007, covered 587 villages out of 669 villages with a population of 1,78,030.
3. Third Round General spray commenced from, 01.09.2007 to 20.11.2007, covered 644 villages out of 669 villages with a population of 2,39,880.
4. Weekly Anti Larval Operations commenced from 01.06.2007 in all villages of the Agency area and Sub Plan area, and conducted Anti Larval Operations effected in the entire district as Dengue cases.
5. Focal spray with Malathion 25 per cent under way conducting to the detected positives of both Agency and Sub Plan area villages.
6. Fogging and Prethrurn sprayings are under way conducting in the villages effected for Malaria, Chikunguniya and Dengue cases in the district.
7. Gambusia Fish is being introduced in the water stagnations of the Agency and Sub Plan areas as routine process.
8. Laboratory services are being strengthened by filling of all Agency area PHCs including newly sanctioned PHCs with Medical Lab Technicians.
9. The required Adulticides, Larvicides, Anti Malarials, etc., are available to meet any emergency in the district.
10. All the Medical Officers are alerted to take up the surveillance of Dengue, Chikunguniya and Japanese Encephalitis cases in the district for early detection of the cases and prompt control measures to arrest the spread of the disease.
11. 48,000 Mosquito nets received and distributed; 27,935 Bed nets to all PHCs of the Agency area.
12. Rapid diagnosis kits distributed to interior villages for spot Blood smears examination through all Medical Officers of the PHCs in the Agency area.
13. E. Mal Injections and Quinine injections supplied to the Agency area PHCs for immediate treatment.
14. Combi-pack (PF treatment) supplied to all PHCs in the Agency area for adult dose.
15. Every 45 days conducting Focal spray with Malathion 25 per cent in the Agency area Hostels and Ashram Schools.
16. Every case village conducting Focal spray, Pyrethrurn spray, Anti Larval Operation and Fogging Operations conducting in November onwards.

17. 60 Jathara Programmes conducted for awareness of Vector born diseases in the Agency area.
18. IEC materials i.e., Dengue calendars, Spiral books, Pamphlets, Dengue charts, CDs and cassettes are distributed in the Primary Health Centres in East Godavari District.

Diseases afflicting the tribals mostly are related to their poverty. Malnutrition is most conspicuous in this context among many tribal communities. Lack of clean drinking water coupled with their cultural practices contribute to many water borne diseases like gastro-enteritis, cholera, etc. Socio-cultural factors assume importance in explaining the etiology, transmission and treatment of the diseases among the tribals not only of Eastern Ghats but elsewhere also. In an earlier study conducted (Rajpramukh, 1998) among the tribals of Munchingput in Visakhapatnam District of Andhra Pradesh the following diseases were found to afflict the tribals as give in Table 5.1

Table 5.1: Prevalence of Various Diseases among the Tribals of Visakhapatnam District during 1983-86

S. No.	*Type of Diseases*	*No. of Cases Reported*	*Average per Year*	*Proportion (%)*
1.	Skin disease	1,69,205	42,301	23.28
2.	Anaemia	1,31,889	32,972	18.14
3.	Arthritis	74,995	18,749	10.32
4.	Malnutrition	72,133	18,033	9.92
5.	Malaria	15,213	3,803	2.09
6.	Eye diseases	10,769	2,692	1.48
7.	Acute respiratory	8,424	2,106	1.16
8.	Peptic ulcer	7,921	1,980	1.09
9.	Ancylostomiasis	7,910	1,978	1.09
10.	Diseases of Teeth	5,036	1,259	0.69
11.	All other diseases	2,23,442	55,861	30.74
	Total	**7,26,936**	**1,81,734**	**100.00**

The total new cases reported during the years 1983 and 1986 (4 years) were 1,83,452 and forms an average of 10.5 per cent of the total population. In other words, about 10 per cent of the total population fall sick every year. Table 5.1 gives 10 major diseases among the tribals during 1983-86 with their corresponding prevalence rate.

Skin Disease: It tops the list of diseases among the tribals. The most commonly reported skin disease among them is scabies which is caused by the itch mite (*sacoptes scabei*). The female mite burrows into the skin and lays eggs causing intense itching which is usually worse at night. Transmission of mites occurs by close body contact and by infected clothes. Among the tribals, unhygienic habits, lack of adequate water facilities and crowded housing are probably responsible for the spread of infection.

Arthritis: This is another major disease prevalent among the tribals. Osteo-arthritis and Rheumatoid arthritis are most common while gout, tuberculous arthritis and suppurative arthritis are less common among them. Osteo-arthritis is mostly seen in the older age-group. This essentially is a 'wear and tear' phenomenon also designated as joint disease characterized by progressive deterioration and loss of cartilage over the years. Rheumatoid arthritis is more prevalent among the females than males, with peak prevalence in third to fourth decades of one's life. It is basically an inflammatory disease of unknown etiology.

Malnutrition: Among the tribals, it is probably due to poverty and ignorance, acute and chronic illness, chronic alcoholism, gastro-intestinal disorders; and diets lacking proteins, vitamin B_{12} and iron. Milk consumption is not practiced by the tribals of Visakhapatnam District, which, if adapted, could have had desirable affects on their health status. Of all these factors among the tribals 'alcoholism' is a behavioural factor which assumes significance in the context of malnutrition.

Malaria: It is endemic almost all over India and the tribal areas are not an exception to it. It is caused due to infection with *sporozoan* parasite of the genus *plasmodium* and transmitted to man by infected female *anopheles* mosquito. Open drainages and unhygienic surroundings serve as breeding places for mosquitoes which are the major environmental factor among the tribals too. As a preventive measure, long sleeves and trousers are advocated. But the tribals dress usually covers their private parts only making large parts of their body exposed to mosquito bites. Non-availability of prophylactic drugs also could be another reason for the prevalence of the disease. However, the high incidence of sickle cell among the tribals makes malaria less severe. But if such cases go unnoticed and the standard regimen for malaria applied to such patients it would prove to be fatal.

Eye Diseases: Of the two eye diseases, trachoma and cataract, trachoma is caused due to the unhygienic conditions. It is a specific communicable kerato conjunctivitis caused by *Chlamydia trachoma*. Transmission is usually by contact or from *fomites* in unhygienic surroundings. Some infections also occur during birth from infected genital passages. Unhygienic surroundings, lack of proper care of the eyes could be easily said to be the causative factors. Lack of trachoma clinics in tribal areas also contribute to the high incidence.

Respiratory Disease: Some of the respiratory diseases among the tribals are chickenpox, influenza, diphtheria, whooping cough and tuberculosis. These respiratory infections are caused by virus and bacteria. Among many tribals some of these respiratory diseases are caused by excessive alcoholism and smoking.

Peptic Ulcer and other Digestive Disorders: These are usually common in middle aged to older adults. The term 'peptic ulcer' refers to an ulcer in the lower esophagus, stomach or duodenum. An increased serum level of calcium stimulates gastric secretion and, therefore, acid secretion in the stomach. Patients with peptic ulcer often have a family history of the disease. Individuals of blood group "O" are about 36 per cent more likely to develop these lesions than those of the other blood groups. Males are more susceptible to peptic ulcer. It is caused due to exposure of duodenal mucosa to excessive amounts of acid and peptin and some breakdown in gastric mucosal defense against acid and peptin. Women are most often affected at, or after, menopause. Smoking usually exacerbates the course of peptic ulcer disease and excessive alcoholism is also bad. The tribal diet which contains sour gruel and rice beer may also contribute to the disease.

Ancylostomiasis: It is caused by the hookworm. As hookworms suck blood it results in anaemia. Worm inhabits duodenum and upper jejunum. Eggs are passed in stools, hatch in moist soil and produce larvae which can penetrate bare feet and reinfect people. Prevention is by wearing shoes and using latrines. As the tribals defecate in the open and not in the habit of wearing shoes, Ancylostomiasis spreads unchecked and is one of the major causes of anaemia among the tribals.

Diseases of Teeth: Many of the teeth disorders among the tribals are caused mostly due to their lack of oral hygiene and smoking habits. In addition, it is found that the water that is available in tribal areas lacks such minerals like iodine and fluoride. In such cases supply of iodized salt to the tribals and usage of fluoride tooth pastes in general would contain some tooth disorders. This is not practiced by many tribals due to non-availability, lack of awareness and as they are non-customary. The social-cultural factors cited for each disease are only suggestive but not conclusive.

Table 5.2: Diseases reported at PHC, Ananthagiri (November-December 2006)

S. No.	Diseases	November. 2006	December 2006
1.	Fevers	90 cases	35 cases
2.	Scabies	60 cases	25 cases
3.	Gastroenteritis	50 cases	20 cases
4.	URTI	35 cases	10 cases
5.	Diarrhoea	20 cases	10 cases
6.	Malaria	15 cases	8 cases
7.	Tuberculosis	10 cases	3 cases
8.	Snake bite	3 cases	2 cases
9.	Mumps	3 cases	–
10.	White discharge	2 cases	–

Source: PHC OP Register.

In another study conducted on the Bondos of Malkangiri District in Orissa Jhansi Rani (2009) reports the diseases afflicting them (Table 5.3).

It can be seen from Table 5.3 that the major group of diseases affecting health status of the studied population is fevers, accidents, cuts and injuries, digestive disorders, cough, eye infection, skin disease, other, E.N.T. disease, muscular disorders and disorder of joints. Fever occupies the highest percentage (29.62). Among other disease group's accident, cuts and injuries (17.58%), digestive disorders (13.72%) cold and cough (13.34%) and infection (9.8%) are very prominent.

According to her study the entire block (Khairput) area is known for endemic malaria. According to the blood slide examination report of the Khairput PHC during the year 2006-2007, one-third of the fever cases were malarial parasite positive cases. Since the Bondo are habituated to smoking and taking tobacco, many of them suffer from prolonged respiratory diseases like pharyngitis and bronchitis. In the long run, pharyngitis leads to Rheumatoid arthritis. People are suffering from night blindness and other deficiency diseases due to deficiency of Vit-A, protein. Further,

Table 5.3: Incidence of Different Diseases and Treatment among the Bondos in 2006-2007

S. No.	*Name of the Disease*	*Total*	*%*	*Treatment*
1.	Fever	537	29.62	Traditional/allopathic/ayurveda
2.	Accident, cuts and injuries	178	8.58	Allopathic
3.	Digestive disorders	295	13.72	Traditional
4.	Cough	287	13.34	Traditional/ayurveda
5.	Eye infection	211	9.81	Allopathic
6.	Skin disease	381	3.76	Traditional/ayurveda
7.	Others	71	3.30	Traditional/allopathic
8.	E.N.T. disease	62	2.88	Allopathic
9.	Muscular disorder	61	2.83	Allopathic
10.	Disorders of joints	60	2.79	Allopathic
11.	Vitamin deficiency	4	0.18	Nil
12.	Senility	1	0.04	Traditional
13.	Diseases of circulatory system	1	0.04	Traditional/allopathic
14.	Other clear symptoms	1	0.04	Allopathic
	Total	**2150**	**100**	

many Bondos suffer from skin diseases due to their unsanitary living habits. Again due to the habit of taking excessive alcohol and other intoxicated drinks, their liver gets damaged and the Bondo suffer from hepatitis and gastritis. Besides the above, a good number of wounded/injury cases are reported most of which are caused by the very criminal attitude of the Bondo. Further in the jungle of Bondo hills, bears and boars frequently injure the Bondo inhabitants.

A comparison of these tables reveal the major diseases afflicting the tribals as, Scabies, Diarrhoea and Gastroenteritis (both water borne), Cough and Malaria and other fevers. Therefore, it can be noticed that even after almost 25 years the disease pattern has not changed among the tribals.

Jhansi Rani (2009) presents the disease profile of the Bondos according to age and sex with the intensity of different diseases as well as social status and health care towards female. It is observed that fever; diarrhoea and dysentery, cold and cough, skin disease, tuberculosis, wounds, chest pain and joint pain are very prominent between both the sexes. The males have the higher percentage of diarrhoea and dysentery (7.8%), cold and cough (8.6%), skin diseases (3.9%), tuberculosis (3.9%) wounds (2.3%) and chest pain (3.9%) than the females. For males, higher percentage of diarrhoea and dysentery is observed in the age group of 45-64 years (11.1%), which may be due to the digestion problem during old age. On the whole though males record the highest percentage of cold and cough, according to the age group, females in the age group of 45-64 years show the highest percentage (18.6%) of cold and cough. It is noticeable that only males in the age group of 0-14 years and 15-44 years are affected by skin diseases, which could be due to irregular bathing habits and bathing in contaminated water. Tuberculosis shows the highest percentage (8.8%) in the age group of 15-44 years among the males. During investigation it is noticed that mostly the male convicts of 15-44 years of age are affected by TB. From the detailed interview of the TB patients it is observed that mostly they (Bondo males) have been affected by TB from outside (jail) of the community. Chest pain and joint pains are high among males of the age group 15-44 years and such problems are due to their heavy workload at hill slope (*dangar*), cutting of trees to prepare the hill patches and excessive drinking of *salap* (sago palm juice). The incidence of fever is the highest in females. Different gynaecological problems may be the root causes of higher percentage of fever among the females.

From above discussion, it may be inferred that due to more exposure of female with outsiders, long imprisonment, heavy work load during rainy and summer season at wet land and the hill slopes the male are more affected by different diseases.

Cultural Factors in the Etiology of Diseases: It is found in many works that the tribals cultural practices and life-styles significantly contribute to the prevalence of diseases in the tribal areas. Their eating habits including their culinary practices and many institutional aspects play a significant role in the outbreak of diseases. To wean them away from such practices is the task of all those concerned with their health.

Food and Culinary Habits: As many illness episodes among the tribals are poverty related, their food naturally lacks all the vitamins and minerals leading to malnutrition. In addition, their culinary practices also contribute to their sickness. In one of our field trips near Rampachodavaram in the 1990s, we noticed tribals eating chicken for over two/three days cutting a small portion from the raw chicken each time. This practice certainly makes the chicken putrefy and they were found consuming it over a period of two/three days. This is only an example and undercooked food also is quite common among them. Added to this it is too well-known that most of them do not consume milk or milk products. On the otherside an average tribal is an alcoholic and a smoker. In recent times the young boys and some girls are found in the habit of consuming 'pan parag', 'ghutka', khaini, etc., which undoubtedly would leave deleterious effects on their health.

Family: With increased nuclearization of the family, the traditional duties and responsibilities too become weakened. To cite an example, in one of our field trips to Chintapalli we found a tribal moaning lying in the cot with deep cut he had while cutting the tree branches three days ago. There was none to take him to the PHC which was located three kilometres away. If the neighbours attend to him, they lose a day's wages which they cannot afford. Wife and younger children were of no use to him at that time as he was to be carried on the cot to the PHC.

Marriage: It is also found that sexual behaviour also plays a vital role in the etiology and transmission of diseases. Among many of the tribals, there is a high prevalence of pre-marital and extra-marital relationships. For example, among the Porjas of Shrujanapeta, it is reported that young boys of about 13-14 years old indulge in sexual relations even with girls older than their age. It is also reported in some cases that younger boys of 8 or 9 years old also have their own girl friends. In yet another instance, while the sons are still in their tender years, the fathers marry girls on behalf of their sons. While it is beyond the scope of this book to deal in detail with the marital practices and sexual relations prevalent among these tribals, it becomes necessary here to touch upon some salient features of their sexual life as they pose health problems of unmanageable proportion. It is reported, as the average Porja is drawn into sexual life at an early age and is constantly engaged in it, by the time they reach 30 or 35 years age, they all become old and eventually die at a relatively younger age. The loose sexual code of conduct among some of the tribals is taken advantage of by the outsiders. For instance, after a battalion of Reserve Police were posted in Munchingput to contain the Naxalite problem in 1990, there was a rapid increase in the sexually transmitted diseases reported at the Munchingput PHC. Problems of this kind could be easily controlled if necessary precautions are taken in checking the contact between tribals and others. High prevalence of polygyny was reported in our recent field work on the Konda Kammaras near Paderu.

Economic Activities: Most of them subsist on cultivation including podu. Many tribals are found working on an average only half-days in a week. If they earn money for two or three days the remaining days they skip work enjoying liquor and slumber.

Political Activities: The benefits of developmental programmes are found in many areas to have been cornered only by the elite among them. In case of Visakhapatnam, only Bhagathas and Valmikis, one at the top of traditional hierarchy and the other at the bottom, have improved their stock leaving behind all others without any significant change.

Gender based Disadvantage: Many tribal women in many parts of Eastern Ghats are found to be anaemic and suffering from malnutrition. Even at the time of eating food, women eat only after all the household members had it. This is a cultural practice among many of the tribes found in this study too. In such a practice by the time it is the turn of the women more often than not they are left with food in sufficient quantity. This is one of the reasons for their being anaemic besides lack of micronutrients in the foods they consume.

Lack of Awareness: In a study conducted among the tribes of Visakhapatnam District in 2009 (R.S. Rao), it was found out that the tribals are not receiving treatment from the PHCs/Malaria Sub-units. Only the Community Health Worker (CHW) is available at the village level and adequate awareness regarding the treatment was not available. It was also pointed in the study that most of the tribal houses are not suitable for bed-nets. Malaria is persistent in many villages because of improper surveillance and also due to the unique forest eco system. It was also mentioned in the study that periodic insecticidal spraying was not reported in all the villages studied.

Some other Statistics: In another study on KAP regarding RCH care among the tribes of Vizianagaram District in 2008 (R.S. Rao) the crude birth rate was reported as 465.27; crude death rate as 28.65; Total number of anti-natal check ups 56.4 per cent; No ANC 2.7 per cent; T.T. 96.5 per cent; No TT 3.1 per cent IFA tablets received 97.3 per cent; Consumed IFA 89.2 per cent; Institutional Deliveries 15.5 per cent; Home Deliveries 84.5 per cent; Birth attendant: Old Women—42.5 per cent; Traditional *dai*—31.5 per cent; Breast Feeding initiation within hour after births—64.2 per cent; Pre-lacteal feeding given 26.7 per cent; Exclusive Breast feeding 8.04 per cent (mostly); Full Immunization 98.1 per cent; Partial Immunization 1.7 per cent; No Immunization 0.2 per cent;

Diarrhoea (Children) 22.7; Pregnancy Complications 75.2 per cent; Delivers Complications 16.87 per cent; Post-natal Complications 16.8 per cent; Abnormal Vaginal discharge 8.1 per cent; Evaluation of Universal Immunization Programme in Tribal areas of Vizianagaram District 2009: Fully immunized—the children under 2 years provided with seven vaccines and Vitamin A supplementation are 66.00 per cent; Partially immunized—the children under 2 years, who missed one or two doses or more vaccines, except booster doses are 33.78 per cent; BCG vaccine—to prevent tuberculosis the BCG vaccine will be provided to new born is 100 per cent; DPT vaccine—the coverage for diphtheria, pertussis and Tetanus in the present population is 74.17 per cent; Measles—in the present study the percentage of measles vaccine coverage is 89.40 per cent only because for two months the measles vaccination was postponed; Polio militias coverage is not satisfactory and is limited to 78.81 per cent; Hepatitis-B—this is one of the common health problems in the study area and the vaccine against hepatitis virus is recently introduced and the coverage should be improved more than 68.87 per cent.

Water Borne Diseases among the Tribals

Water is the prime sustaining element for life on earth. The linkage between safe drinking water and health and productivity of human beings is well established. Hence, the manner of utilization of water and its disposal have a close bearing on the morbidity and mortality of human beings. Safe drinking water could make a tremendous impact on the quality of life in our villages, because availability of safe drinking water has direct impact on the working conditions and health of the people and their productive capacity. It has been noticed that the problem of supply of potable drinking water to different tribal village is very complex and challenging.

The prevalence of water borne disease is very high among the tribals. This high prevalence is usually due to certain behavioural practices and the quality of drinking water. Bore well water is usually considered safe as compared to river or open well water. In an earlier study (Elizabeth *et al.*, 2000) drinking water samples of bore wells from Gangannadoravalasa and Reddavalasa tribal villages of Vizianagram District in Andhra Pradesh were analysed. Microbiological analysis of these water samples showed high coliform and high total plate counts. These results indicate high contamination of these waters with pathogenic microorganisms, thereby causing frequent fevers, diarrhoea, dysentery and gastroenteritis.

It is too well known that almost all human settlements lie nearby a water point. In the agency area each tribal settlement is usually situated near a hill stream (*gedda)* or spring (*oota neeru).* The tribal people in this area refer to any type of water resource as Ganga (sacred water) and it has religious significance.

According to the 1991 census, Vizianagaram District in Andhra Pradesh has a tribal population of 1,52,335 which is 7.8 per cent of the total district population. The predominant tribes of the district are: Jatapus, Savaras, Konda doras, Mooka doras, Manne doras and Gadabas. Gangannadoravalasa, a plains villages and Reddavalasa, a hill top village are two tribal villages of Vizianagram District inhabited by Konda dora and Jatapu/savara tribals respectively. Both the villages come under Pachipenta Primary Health Centre.

The results of the study indicated that the bore well waters of Gangannadora Valasa and Redda Valasa were highly contaminated with microbes and the high prevalence of morbidity among the tribals of these two villages obviously could be related to the regular consumption of these contaminated waters. In the present study though their drinking waters are drawn from the bore wells, their practice of open defecation or dumping human and animal excreta near the bore wells might have caused the bacteria to leach and pollute the ground water. The hardness, fluorides iron content in the waters of Gangannadora Valasa were very high when compared to those of Redda Valasa villages suggesting that the Redda Valasa water is more potable than that of Gangannadora Valasa Village. The chemical toxicity of water may also be responsible for the poor health of these villagers.

As the physico-chemical properties cannot be changed easily, it is advisable for the tribals to boil and cool the water before consumption. Boiling water helps to kill microbes and cooling helps settling of minerals like, calcium, magnesium, etc., and also remove some of the hardness.

In another study of this kind by the same authors the microbiological and physico-chemical parameters of drinking water samples from two villages of Vizianagaram District were monitored. The microbiological analysis of Janjavathi river water showed very high faecal coliform counts and large number of colony forming units (cfu) i.e., 540/100 ml and 2.18×10^8/ml as determined by MPN test and standard total plate count methods respectively. Borewell water from Sominaiduvalasa village showed 1600 coliforms per 100 ml sample and 4.3×10^9 cfu/ml, indicating that these waters are highly polluted with microbial pathogens. Therefore, the water is non-potable. Physico-chemical parameters such as pH, conductivity, Total Solids (TS), Total Dissolved Solids (TDS), total hardness, Calcium hardness, Magnesium hardness, Chlorides, Fluorides, Sulphates and Iron were beyond the permissible limits in bore well water indicating that this water is non-potable.

High incidence of water borne diseases, viz., gastroenteritis, amoebiasis, bacillary dysentery and occasional cholera among the tribals could be partly due to their unhygienic water which possess higher amounts of minerals and other pathogenic microorganisms than the permissible limits. As the quality of drinking water available in Vizianagaram sub-plan area has not been scientifically established so far, it is conceived in this study to collect drinking water samples from various sources like springs, rivers, bore wells and conduct microbiological, physico-chemical tests. Accordingly results obtained from the villages are presented here.

The results of this study too indicated that both the river as well as the bore water are highly polluted with pathogenic microorganisms, through faecal contamination as judged by high coliform counts and total plate counts. Regarding the high counts in bore water, there may be open defecation or dumping yards near the bore well and the coliforms might have leached into the ground waters causing microbiological pollution which ultimately leads to various water borne diseases. The total hardness, magnesium hardness, chlorides, total dissolved solids and iron content are very high in bore water than the river water. The people should drink boiled water which may eliminate microbiological and chemical pollution of water to some extent. But the toxic effects caused by heat stable toxins of pathogens cannot be removed by drinking boiled water.

In a study conducted among the tribes of Visakhapatnam District in 2009 (R.S. Rao), it was found that the tribals are not receiving treatment from the PHCs/Malaria Sub-units. Only the Community Health Worker (CHW) is available at the village level and adequate awareness regarding the treatment was not available.

It was also pointed out in the study that most of the tribal houses are not suitable for bed-nets. Malaria is persistent in many villages because of improper surveillance and also due to the unique forest eco system. It was also mentioned in the study that periodic insecticidal spraying was not reported in all the villages studied.

AIDS/HIV: Today AIDS is the third biggest killer in the world. According to UNAIDS, at the end of 2004, 42 million people are living with HIV/AIDS and there were 5.13 million new infections and 3.1 million deaths occurred. If we look at the global scenario, every day 14,000 new infections occur. Of these 2,000 infections were among those below 14 years age (primarily through vertical transmission). Out of the 12,000 infections occurring in the age group of 15 years and above, 50 per cent of infections (i.e., 6000) occur in the age group of 15-24 years placing the young people in the centre of the epidemic.

HIV estimates for India grew enormously since 1990. In, 1990 it was 0.2 million and by 1994 it went up to 1.7 million. In 1998 it was 3.5 million and by 2000 it went up to 3.86 million. For 2001, it was 3.97 million while it was 4.58 million in 2002 and in 2003 it reached 5.1 million. Nearly 80 per cent of people with HIV/AIDS in South Asia are in India and the reasons for such a high prevalence could be traced to a host of socio-economic, cultural and biological factors. Andhra Pradesh is one of the top three States in India in registering highest number of HIV/AIDS cases only next to Maharashtra and Tamilnadu.

HIV Prevalence in Andhra Pradesh: At the end of 2004, the estimate for HIV positive people in Andhra Pradesh (India) is 5.68 lakhs, which is almost 1/10 of the national figure. Of the 23 districts in Andhra Pradesh, 17 districts reported 1 per cent HIV positive, 12 districts reported 2 per cent and above among the pregnant women, 92 per cent of the infected are in the age group of 15-49 years and 88.5 per cent of the infections were through sexual route of transmission. Other modes of transmissions (3.64%) include parents to child transmissions; infected syringes (0.99%); Blood and blood products (0.96%); and others (5.90%).

Conditions for Rapid Growth of HIV in Andhra Pradesh: About one in five men report non-regular sexual partners and the sexually transmitted infections are 7 per cent in both male and female. Another reason is the low rate of condoms use. Large migrant population also contributes to the rapid growth of HIV with increasing trafficking of girls into sex trade. Existence of strong traditional sexual networks having links to Mumbai, Goa and Pune and vast network of national highways are the other reason.

Along side the international effort towards a more comprehensive scientific view of the epidemic and general availability of medical treatment, information/education/communication (IEC) is a key instrument in the efficient prevention and support to infected and sick people in the perspective of sustainable human development. In order to give it full significance and long-term effects, it has to be elaborated and developed within the context of the cultural approach. In other words, the validity of ICE is and will be tested through the response of population that will result either in continuity or change in their ways of thinking, value systems and styles of life in relation to the epidemic. Who could be better than an Anthropologist to handle such a situation as the key concept in anthropology is 'Culture'? An Anthropologist's participant observation method makes him eventually a member of the community while doing field work and evidently he would be able to convincingly talk to people in changing their life styles, ways of thinking and value systems, with the ultimate goal to define conditions for their sensitization and mobilization in prevention and care. In addition, valuable IEC activity can work effectively with the collaboration of an Anthropologist with analyzing in-depth specific characters of target audiences, identifications and segmentation of the various "risk group" in their cultural relations with socio-economic development and general society. The culture approach means that any given population's culture reference and resources, such as way of life, value system, traditions and beliefs and the fundamental human rights, will be considered as key references in building a framework for strategies and project planning. These key references will also serve as the resources and basics for building a relevant response and sustainable action in prevention and care as well as in impact reduction. This becomes an indispensable condition to achieve in-depth and long-term changes in people's behaviour and to give full consistency to medical and sanitary strategies. Thus the cultural approach to AIDS and drug abuse problem as well is the best suited method and Anthropologists are well equipped to handle the situation. A case study of HIV/AIDS Prevention Programmes in East Godavari District is given in Table 5.4 to 5.9 including some areas that cover tribal population.

Table 5.4: Performance of ICTCs in Agency Area in East Godavari District for the Period of April '2006 to March 2007

S. No.	*Name of the Centre*		*VCTC Component*		*PPTCT Component*									
		Targets upto March – 2007	*Total Tested*	*Total Positives*	*Total ANCs Registered*	*Total Tested*	*Total Positives*	*Total +ve Deliveries*	*Total Live Births for +ve Women*	*Total MB Pairs Received NVP*	*Total Tests Conducted*	*Achievement %*	*Total Positives*	*Positivity Percentage*
1.	CHC, Rampachodavaram	1200	284	12	0	0	0	0	0	0	284	23.67	12	4.23
2.	GH, Addateegala	600	362	18	619	615	7	2	1	1	977	162.83	25	2.56
3.	PHC, Maredumilli	500	293	5	151	151	3	1	0	0	444	88.80	8	1.80
4.	CHC, Y. Ramavaram	500	304	6	109	109	5	1	1	1	413	82.60	11	2.66
5.	PHC, Rajavommangi	500	322	18	300	300	3	0	0	0	622	124.40	21	3.38
	Total	**3300**	**1565**	**59**	**1179**	**1175**	**18**	**4**	**2**	**2**	**2740**	**83.03**	**77**	**2.81**
		VCTC Positivity			3.77									
		PPTCT Positivity			1.53									

Table 5.5: Performance of ICTCs in Agency Area in East Godavari District for the Period of April '2007 and March' 2008

S. No.	*Name of the Centre*	*Targets upto March – 2008*	*VCTC Component*		*PPTCT Component*						*Total Tests Conducted*	*Achievement %*	*Total Positives*	*Positivity Percentage*
			Total Tested	*Total Positives*	*Total ANCs Registered*	*Total Tested*	*Total Positives*	*Total +ve Deliveries*	*Total Live Births for +ve Women*	*Total MB Pairs Received NVP*				
1.	CHC, Rampachodavaram	1000	1184	48	454	341	2	0	0	0	1525	152.50	50	3.28
2.	GH, Addateegala	500	511	18	853	788	6	4	3	3	1299	259.80	24	1.85
3.	PHC, Maredumilli	500	401	9	273	273	0	0	0	0	674	134.80	9	1.34
4.	CHC, Y. Ramavaram	500	478	8	152	152	2	0	0	0	630	126.00	10	1.59
5.	PHC, Rajavommangi	500	544	19	375	428	2	1	1	1	972	194.40	21	2.16
	Total	**3000**	**3118**	**102**	**2107**	**1982**	**12**	**5**	**4**	**4**	**5100**	**170.00**	**114**	**2.24**
		VCTC Positivity			3.27									
		PPTCT Positivity			0.61									

Table 5.6: Performance of ICTCs in Agency Area in East Godavari District for the Period of April '2008 and October' 2008

S. No.	Name of the Centre	Targets upto March-2009	VCTC Component		PPTCT Component						Total Tests Conducted
			Total Tested	*Total Positives*	*Total ANCs Registered*	*Total Tested*	*Total Positives*	*Total +ve Deliveries*	*Total Live Births for +ve Women*	*Total MB Pairs Received NVP*	
1.	CHC, Rampachodavaram	2000	717	41	453	639	2	0	0	0	1170
2.	GH, Addateegala	1000	213	6	645	410	1	0	0	0	623
3.	PHC, Maredumilli	1000	229	6	186	186	0	0	0	0	415
4.	CHC, Y.Ramavaram	1000	277	7	174	169	1	0	0	0	861
5.	PHC, Rajavommangi	1000	181	16	314	396	1	3	3	3	577
	Total	**6000**	**1617**	**76**	**1772**	**1800**	**5**	**3**	**3**	**3**	**3646**
	VCTC Positivity	4.70	Higher % is due to Scarcity in HIV Testing Kits during January to March '2008								
	PPTCT Positivity	0.28									

Table 5.7: Integrated Testing and Counselling Centres: Performance of ICTCs in Agency Area in East Godavari District for the Period of April '2006 to March' 2007

S. No.	Name of the Centre	Targets upto March 2007	VCTC Component		PPTCT Component									
			Total Tested	Total Positives	Total ANCs Registered	Total Tested	Total Positives	Total +ve Deliveries	Total Live Births for +ve Women	Total MB Pairs Received NVP	Total Tests Conducted	Achievement %	Total Positives	Positivity %
1.	CHC, Rampachodavaram	1200	284	12	0	0	0	0	0	0	284	23.67	12	4.23
2.	GH, Addateegala	600	362	18	619	615	7	2	1	1	977	162.83	25	2.56
3.	PHC, Maredumilli	500	293	5	151	151	3	1	0	0	444	88.80	8	1.80
4.	CHC, Y. Ramavaram	500	304	6	109	109	5	1	1	1	413	82.60	11	2.66
5.	PHC, Rajavommangi	500	322	18	300	300	3	0	0	0	622	124.40	21	3.38
	Total	3300	1565	59	1179	1175	18	4	2	2	2740	83.03	77	2.81
		VCTC positivity			3.77									
		PPTCT Positivity			1.53									

Table 5.8: Performance of ICTCs in Agency Area in East Godavari District for the Period of April '2007 and March' 2008

S. No.	Name of the Centre	Targets upto March –2008	VCTC Component		PPTCT Component									
			Total Tested	Total Positives	Total ANCs Registered	Total Tested	Total Positives	Total +ve Deliveries	Total Live Births for +ve Women	Total MB Pairs Received NVP	Total Tests Conducted	Achievement %	Total Positives	Positivity %
1.	CHC, Rampachodavaram	1000	1184	48	454	341	2	0	0	0	1525	152.50	50	3.28
2.	GH, Addateegala	500	511	18	853	788	6	4	3	3	1299	259.80	24	1.85
3.	PHC, Maredumilli	500	401	9	273	273	0	0	0	0	674	134.80	9	1.34
4.	CHC, Y.Ramavaram	500	478	8	152	152	2	0	0	0	630	126.00	10	1.59
5.	PHC, Rajavommangi	500	544	19	375	428	2	1	1	1	972	194.40	21	2.16
	Total	**3000**	**3118**	**102**	**2107**	**1982**	**12**	**5**	**4**	**4**	**5100**	**170.00**	**114**	**2.24**
		VCTC positivity			3.27									
		PPTCT Positivity			0.61									

Table 5.9: Performance of ICTCs in Agency Area in East Godavari District for the Period of April '2008 and October '2008

S. No.	Name of the Centre	Targets upto March – 2009	VCTC Component		PPTCT Component						Total Tests Conducted	Achievement %	Total Positives	Positivity Percentage
			Total Tested	Total Positives	Total ANCs Registered	Total Tested	Total Positives	Total +ve Deliveries	Total Live Births for +ve Women	Total MB Pairs Received NVP				
1.	CHC, Rampachodavaram	2000	717	41	453	639	2	0	0	0	1170	58.50	43	3.68
2.	GH, Addateegala	1000	213	6	645	410	1	0	0	0	623	62.30	7	1.12
3.	PHC, Maredumilli	1000	229	6	186	186	0	0	0	0	415	41.50	6	1.45
4.	CHC, Y.Ramavaram	1000	277	7	174	169	1	0	0	0	861	86.10	8	0.93
5.	PHC, Rajavommangi	1000	181	16	314	396	1	3	3	3	577	57.70	17	2.95
	Total	**6000**	**1617**	**76**	**1772**	**1800**	**5**	**3**	**3**	**3**	**3646**	**60.77**	**81**	**2.22**
		VCTC Positivity		4.70	Higher % is due to Scarcity in HIV Testing Kits during January to March '2008									
		PPTCT Positivity		0.28										

PPTCT= *Prevention of Parent to Child Transmission;* VCTC= *Voluntary Counselling and Testing Centres.*

VI

Tribal Ethno-Medicine

Field researches in different parts of India have yielded a rich body of data on tribal ethno-medicine. The local medicine man usually administers these herbal medicines besides treating diseases dealing with supernatural beings. Some of the tribals too are well versed in the medicinal properties of these herbs available in their forest eco-system.

Medicinal plants constitute an integral part of indigenous, folk and tribal medical system. The Irulas and Paniyas are two of the six tribes inhabiting Nilgiris. These groups rely on superstitions and supernatural elements. They attribute bodily disorders to the metaphysical forces. Magico-religious practices form an integral part of their ethno-medicine.

According to the Irulas, they are good at treating snake bites, dog bites and headache by magico-religious methods. For example the juice of drum stick leaves (*Moringa oleifera*) is used by them to cure scorpion bite and curiously if the bite is on the left side the juice is poured in the right ear and *vice-versa*. They believe that epidemics are caused by the anger of gods. They appease them with fowl and goat sacrifices.For them measles are due to the violation of social taboos. Both Paniyas and Irulas consider Papaya *(Caric papay)* fruit as hot and abortifacient hence avoid during pregnancy. Further pregnant women are forbidden to eat brinjal (*Solanum melangena*)(egg plant) as it is believed to cause skin problems to the new born. Tomoto (*Lycopersicon lycopersicum*) is considered cold hence avoided during pregnancy among the Irulas. The pregnant women among them are given Tamarind juice

(*Tamarindus indica*) in the form of *rasam* (cooked juice) to enhance milk secretion (Rajan *et al.* 2007: 259-270).

In the Visakhapatnam agency area of Andhra Pradesh different herbal medicines are used for various illnesses. For example, in Araku valley a small plant, *kukkuru mutha* (*Elephantopus scaber*) root is used to make a decoction and this is administered to patients suffering from joint pains. Among the Porjas, a small herb, *'pedda loyi'*, (*Eupharbia nirifolia*) is used for different purposes. For eye infections the milk of this herb mixed with ash is applied. This treatment also is given to their animals. This application is also administered for back ache. The Shaman in Gudem Kotha Veedhi, a tribal village, administers two doses of the ground root of *'seema theega'*, (*'Sisampalus pareera'*) mixed with water for treating throat pain and constipation. Among the Khonds a fern, *Rama bhanam* (*Hemonitis arifolia*) leaf is ground with water and is given to those suffering from cough. When taken with milk it rejuvenates the patient with new vigour. In East Godavari District among the tribals, wild onion (*Argenia indica*) is widely used to treat lesions and boils. It is ground into a fine paste and applied to hair to get rid of lice. The bark of *'Billa chettu'* (*Chlorozytis sweetinia*) is used for stomach pain. The root of *Kasivinda (Kesia occidentalis)* with the root of turmeric (*Curcuma longa*) is given in three doses to treat white discharge (*leucaria*) among the women. For snake bites, the root of *pathala garuda* (*Rawulfia radeshng)* together with the roots of *sahadevi (Verninia synera)* and *nalla easwari (Arishtalokhia indica)* is ground into fine powder and a decoction is made with black peppers and orally administered to the patient hourly 10 ml. One most important thing to be observed by those who are present there is while the patient is being treated no one should smoke cigars around that place.

Among the Savaras and Jatapus of Srikakulam district the Yejjodu (Shaman) uses different roots like *jogigirada (Clirodendrum serretum), vepa patta (Ajada raktha), naga saram (Arishtalokhia indica)* for worm infestations in children. For colds, powdered *kukkoti* seeds (*Cleom viscoja)* are used. Besides the magician some among the Savaras and Jatapus have the knowledge related to herbal medicine. They identify the male and female species on the basis of the quantum of production. The tree which gives more production is considered female and the one which gives less production is male. This idea conceptualizes the females as more productive in the realm of reproduction. The following medicinal plants are used by the tribals for the illnesses mentioned against them: *Vusiri (Embilica officionalis)* for body pains; *Nallajeedi (Semicarpus anacardium)* for cough; *Gannery (Thevitia peruvina)* for wounds; *Pukejam (Leucas cephalstus)* for pains; *Gantham (Santhalum albus)* for head aches; *Ankudu (Ficus* species) for wounds; *Karakkai (Terminalia chebula)* for cough and cold; *Tutibodda (Lamblogyn)* for bone fracture; *Osendra* for gastric problems; *Rakasi* for eye diseases; *Rambalam (Annona squamosa)* for abortion and menstrual disorders; *Tulasi (Oscimum sanctum)* for cough and cold; the extractions from such leaves of *dasari, jammi, thangedu* and *kanuga* including garlic are used for abortions; *Nalleru* for paralysis and *Magasirigedda* for impotence.

Among the Konda Reddy, Koyas and Valmikis of West Godavari District, the *Vadde* or *Vaidyakudu* (the medicine man or shaman) uses the bark of *Oodugumanu (Elangium salvifolium)* for cough as an expectorant. For body pains the barks of *Anem* tree *(Bridelia rituza), bhootha vegisa (Kesine glouca), garugudu (Garuga pinneta), uciri manu (Phyllanthus emblica)* are used.

Among the Konda Doras of Vizianagaram, the Shaman uses the barks of *Kothi korandam (Mymoja rubikoulis), gotti (Jijifus zylopyrus), parimi (Jijifus enoplia), billa (Chlorozylan sweetinia)* for pains in the waist and legs. Shankar Rao (2008) gives a list of medicinal plants cultivated on commercial level in the agency areas inhabited by Savaras and Jatapus in Vizianagaram District (*see* Table 6.1).

Hemadri's (1994) work on the tribal medicine in coastal Andhra districts is a very interesting and significant contribution and for further references his account gives an elaborate understanding of the tribal medicine in Andhra Pradesh.

Hemant Bag and Kapoor (2007: 37-38) reports the following diseases during the last six months of their study in this order: Malaria/fever (31.33%); Cough (21.15%); Dysentery (9.14%); Headache (8.09%); Small Pox (5.22%); Typhoid (4.43%) Dental Pain; (3.92%); Sore Eyes (3.66%); Scabies (3.39%); and other minor ailments. They seek both traditional and modern means of treatment. Females play an important role in home remedies among the Kondhs. *Karanj* leaf and custard oil are applied for boils; Saliva is applied for ear pain; If a patient does not get cured within a day or two he/she may be taken to the *Baid, Herbalist, Gunia or Guru* (witch doctor), *pujari*/medical doctor. The following are some of the herbal medicines used by Kondhs for the following diseases:

Table 6.1: Herbal Medicine among the Savaras and Jatapus

S. No.	*Botanical Name of the Plant*	*Telugu*	*Parts*	*Period of Availability*
	(1)	(2)	(3)	(4)
1.	*Abrus precatorius*	*Guruginja*	Roots, leaves & seeds	February-June
2.	*Abutilon indicum*	*Advavi benda*	Whole Plant, leaves, Flowers, Root, Seeds	December-April
3.	*Acacia nitotica ssp. Indica*	*Nalla Tumma*	Bark, Pods, Gum	November – February
4.	*Acacia catechu*	*Kachu, Sandra*	Katha, Bark	
5.	*Achyranthes aspera*	*Apamargamu, Uttareni*	Whole plant, roots, seeds	(Fruits) June-November,
6.	*Actinopteris radiate*	*Mayura sikha*	Whole plant	(seeds) January-May
7.	*Adatoda vasika*	*Addasaramu*	Leaves, Flowers, Roots	October-March
8.	*Aegle marmelos*	*Bilava, Maredu*	Roots, Flowers, Unripe & ripened leaves	October-March
9.	*Aerva lanata*	*Kondapindi, Pindikura*	Whole Plant, Roots, Flowers	
10.	*Albizzia amara*	*Sikireni*	Gum, leaves, seed oil	October-January
11.	*Aloe indica*	*Kalabanda*	Leaf juice	Almost throughout the year
12.	*Alstonia scholas*	*Yedukula ponna*	Bark, latex	
13.	*Andrographis paniculata*	*Nelavemu*	Whole Plant	October-January
14.	*Argemone mexicana*	*Brahmadandi*	Latex, Roots, Seeds, Seed oil	October-April
15.	*Argyreia speciosa*	*Chandra pala, Samudra pala*	Roots, leaves	October-December

(*Contd.*)

(1)	(2)	(3)	(4)
16. *Asparagus racemosus*	*Pilli peechara*	Roots	Throughout the year
17. *Alangium lamarckii*	*Udugu, Ankolam*	Roots, Bark, Leaves, Flowers	May-July
18. *Acacia torta*	*Tella korintha, Konda korintha*	Plant	Throughout the year
19. *Bauhinia purpurea*	*Kanchanam*	Stem, Bark, Roots, Flowers, Buds	September-January
20. *Bocrhaavia diffusa*	*Atikamamidi, Giligeru*	Whole plant, Roots, Leaves	Throughout the year
21. *Bombax malabaricum*	*Mundla Booruga*	Roots, Root Bark, Gum	Throughout the year
22. *Buchanania latifolia*	*Morli, Morlu chettu, Sara*	Leaves, Gum, Seeds	
23. *Butea monosperma*	*Mooduga, Palash*	Gum, Bark, Roots, Leaves, Flowers	(Fruits) February-April, (Seeds April-May
24. *Butea superba*	*Teega moodugu, Kesu*	Leaves, Seeds, Roots, Stem, Seeds	March-May
25. *Caesalpinia bonduc*	*Gatchcha kaya*	Leaves, Bark, Seeds	December-February
26. *Caesalpinia digyna*	*Nune gacha*	Roots	Throughout the year
27. *Caesearia elliptica*	*Girigidi, Chilaka dudduga*	Bark, Fruits	
28. *Calotropis gigantean*	*Jilledu*	Root, Bark, Leaves, Flowers	Almost throughout the year
29. *Canscora deccusata*	*Taripe*	Plant, Juice of plant	June-July
30. *Careya arborea*	*Duddippa, Taripi*	Leaves Bark, Flowers	(Fruits) February-April
31. *Cassia alata*	*Sima avisa*	Leaves	
32. *Cassia angustifolia italica*	*Sunamukhi*	Leaves, Fruits	

(*Contd.*)

(1)	(2)	(3)	(4)
33. *Cassia auriculata*	*Tangedu*	Bark, Leaves, Roots, Seeds	Almost throughout the year
34. *Cassia fistula*	*Rela*	Root, Root bark, Leaves, Flowers, Seeds	August –December
35. *Cassia occidentalis*	*Kasinda*	Whole plant, Roots, Leaves, Seeds	January onwards
36. *Cassia tora*	*Tantemu, Tagirisa*	Roots, Leaves, Seeds	December-April
37. *Catunaregam spinosa*	*Manga*	Bark, Fruit pulp	Almost throughout the year
38. *Celastrus paniculata*	*Malkangini, Jyotishmati*	Bark, Seeds, Seed oil	August –September
39. *Curuculigo orchioides*	*Nelatadigaddalu*	Rhizome	Almost throughout the year
40. *Cycus Circinalis*	*Madana kamakshi*	Bark, Leaves, Seeds	
41. *Cyperus rotundus*	*Tungamusta*	Tubers	Almost throughout the year
42. *Datura alba*	*Ummetha*	Roots, Leaves, Seeds	
43. *Decalepsi hamiltonii*	*Maredugedda*	Roots	November-January
44. *Eclipta alba*	*Gunta Kalagaru Guntagalijeru*	Whole plant, Leaves, Roots	Throughout the year
45. *Euphorbia hirta*	*Reddivarinanubolu*	Whole plant, Latex	Throughout the year
46. *Ficus glomerata*	*Atti, Bodda, Paidi, Udumbaramu*	Bark, Leaves, Flowers, Latex, Roots	March-July
47. *Fluggea microcarpa*	*Purugudu*	Roots, Leaves	Throughout the year
48. *Gloriosa superba*	*Adavi-Nabhi, Pottidumpa*	Tubers	During and after rain
49. *Gmelina arborea*	*Gummadi, Tekugummadi*	Leaves, Flowers, Fruits, Roots, Bark	March-June

(Contd.)

(1)	(2)	(3)	(4)
50. *Gymnema sylvestre*	*Podapatri*	Whole plant, Leaves	Throughout the year except summer
51. *Helicteres Isora*	*Nulitada*	Bark, Fruits, Roots, Root bark	August-December
52. *Hemidesmus indicus*	*Sugandhipala*	Roots	Throughout the year
53. *Holarrhena autidysenterica*	*Kodisapala*	Bark, Seeds	February –July
54. *Centella asiatica*	*Saraswathi*	Whole plant	Throughout the year
55. *Holostemma adakodien*	*Dudipala Teega*	Roots	Throughout the year
56. *Ipomoca maurltiana*	*Nela Gummadi*	Roots	Throughout the year
57. *Jatropha curcas*	*Nepalam*	Leaves, Seeds, Plant Juice	Winter
58. *Jatropha gossypifolia*	*Seema Nepalem*	Leaves, Bark, Seeds	Rainy season
59. *Mangifera indica*			
60. *Mallotus phillippensis*	*Sindhuri, Pandrika*	Powder on the flowers	February-March
61. *Mimosa pudica*	*Peddanidra kanni, Attapatti*	Roots, Leaves, Fruit	Throughout the year
62. *Mucuna prurieus*	*Pilliadugu, Duradagondi*	Roots, Fruits, Seeds	November-February
63. *Myristica fragrans*	*Jaji*		
64. *Ocimum basilicum*	*Rudrajada, Bhutulasi*	Roots, Leaves, Flowers, Seeds	
65. *Ocimum sanctum*	*Tulasi*	Roots, Leaves, Seeds	Throughout the year
66. *Phyllanthus amarus*	*Nela usiri*	Whole plant	
67. *Plumbago rosea, Plumbago Indica*	*Errachitramulam*	Roots, Milky Juice	October-February

(*Contd.*)

(1)	(2)	(3)	(4)
68. *Plumbago zeylanica*	*Tellachitramulam*	Roots, Milky Juice	October-February
69. *Psoralea corylifolia*	*Bavanchalu*	Seeds	
70. *Pueraria tuberose*	*Nela Gummadi, Magagiri gadda*	Tubers	
71. *Rauvolfia serpentine*	*Patalagaridi, Sarpagandhi*	Roots, Leaves	Around December after leaves shedding
72. *Sida cordifolia*	*Bala*	Roots, Leaves, Seeds	October –December
73. *Siegesbekia orientalis*		While plant	
74. *Solanum Xanthocarpum (Solanum Surrentese)*	*Pinnamulaka, Nelamumulaka, Mulla vanga vakudu*	Roots, Plant, Leaves	Almost throughout the year
75. *Sphaeranthus indicus*	*Bodataram, Bobatarupu, Boddasoramu*	Roots, Seeds	November – June
76. *Syzygium cumini*	*Neredu*	Bark, Leaves, Flowers, Seeds	
77. *Terminalia arjuna*	*Naramamudi, Erramamudi, Tellamaddi*	Bark, Twigs, Leaves, Fruits	(Fruits) April-May, June-September
78. *Terminalia belerica*	*Thanikaya*	Bark, Fruits, Oil, Gum	July-October
79. *Tinospora cordifolia*	*Tippateega*	Roots, Leaves, Fruits	October-December
80. *Tragia involucrate*	*Teegaduradagundi, Chinnaduradagondi*	Roots, Leaves, Fruits	May-November
81. *Tribulus terrestris*	*Chinnipalleru*	Roots, Leaves, Fruits	(Fruits) August-October
82. *Trichosanthes cucumerina*	*Chedupotla*	Roots, Leaves, Seeds	Throughout the year

(*Contd.*)

(1)	(2)	(3)	(4)
83. *Ventilago madraspatana*	*Errasurugudu*	Root, Bark	October-April
84. *Vernonia cinerea*	*Sahadevi*	Roots, Plant, Flowers, Seeds	Throughout the year
85. *Withania somnifera*	*Pannerugadda, Aswagandha*	Roots, Leaves, Fruits, Seeds	(Fruit) December, (Roots) January-March
86. *Woodfordia fruticosa*	*Are, Jaji*	Dried Flowers	January-April
87. *Xanthium strumarium*	*Marulamathangi*	Roots, Plant, Fruits	(Plants) July-October, November-December

Source: G.C.C. Visakhapatnam.

1. *Fever/Malaria*: The root of palsa (*Saccharum species*) are powdered and kept in an earthen pot with water for 3-4 hours. About 100 ml of this water is given to the patient thrice a day. Leaf of the pumpkin is boiled in water and the patient is bathed in this water.
2. *Cough*: 2 to 4 grams of roots of Badi Anola, tulsi 'Basil' in equal amount are crushed in Mahu rasa (*Basis latifolia*) and the mixture is given to the patient twice a day. In some cases people keep a piece of root of Badi Anola in the mouth for curing cough.
3. *Scorpion bite*: The roots of Kaincha 'crab eye' plant are rubbed on a stone with water and the paste, applied to the bite. Sometimes the neem (*Azadirachta indica*) nirmuli and satavari leaves are also used to induce vomiting.
4. *Dysentery*: The roots of tatua (*Datura stromium*) are crushed and kept overnight in a pot of water. About 100 ml of this water is given twice a day.
5. *Headache*: The roots of Kadaba (*Zyzyphus jujube*) creeper are crushed with water and applied on the forehead. The leaves of Gutuchta creeper are tied on head.

There are 7 hospitals and 8 PHCs in Kalahandi District. Malaria and cough dominate the number of cases treated at the hospital or PHCs or even by the private medical practitioner.

Behura and Mohanty (2006: 100-143) report the diseases discussed below which are more or less common among the Koya and the Saora as they inhabit similar eco-environment on the Eastern Ghats hill range. The altitude of Koya Territory is relatively less as it constitutes the Godavari basin. Symptoms of the diseases being similar, therapy is not very much dissimilar between them. Broadly they are similar but in detail they are unequal.

1. *Fever*: The Koya call it *edek* and the Saora, *ashu depuno*. The *Wadde* or Shaman (among the Koya), *Kudanboi* or Shamanin (among the Saora) is approached to decipher the cause of suffering. He/She locates the cause through divination and propitiates the concerned spirit through sacrificial rite. The Wadde prescribes the juice of neem (*Azadirachta indica*) leaves to be taken twice a day whereas the Saora shaman administers a mixture of *horida (caparis horida)* and *bahada*

(terminalis balerium) and prescribes spirit sacrificed magico-religious charms to be worn by the patient.

2. *Swelling of the body*: probably caused due to anaemia very common among the Koya who call it *toita*. The Wadde prescribes the juice of *Dimiri* tree (*Ficus glomerata*) root to be taken twice after food.
3. *Swelling of Inngual lymph glands*: The Koyas call it *Gadtul Gada* and the Saora call it *Padaplang*. Symptoms are swelling of lymph glands, rise of body temperature and headache. Koya shaman prescribes hearth cider to be applied over the glands while the Saora medicine man prescribes honey mixed with the juice of *Tulsi (Ocimum sanctum)* leaves to be applied over the swelling.
4. *Malnutrition*: It is known as *Kanchaka* among the Koya. Their belief is that it is due to inadequate food intake as well as by taking or consuming some harmful or noxious food. The shaman prescribes some cashew seed oil to be gently massaged at the naval point of the patient for relief.
5. *Hookworm infestation*: A very common disease among the Koya. The popular belief is that it is due to the intrusion of a spirit into the body. But the allopathic Doctors maintain that it is due to their habit of eating raw pork. The patient experiences pain in the abdomen. The medicine man prescribes an admixture of turmeric paste and neem (*Azadirachta indica)* leaves to be taken orally by the patient once daily before taking food.
6. *Roundworm infestation*: The belief among the Koyas is that it is due to spirit invasion into the body through witchcraft. This disease is known among them as Asapuduku and the medicine-man prescribes 10 gms of turmeric paste to be taken orally twice daily along with a few neem leaves in addition to warding of the spirit through magico-religious rites.
7. *Colic Pain*: It is known as *Dokamandita* among the Koya. This is also believed to have been caused by spirit intrusion. The shaman prescribes a medicine made of sun-dried rice, few strands of a locally available grass called poddaver, ten bits of *rasuna (Alinum sabira),* and a piece of the bark of mango tree (Mangifera indica) to be

administered thrice daily. In addition the shaman performs certain rites to ward off the spirit.

8. *Amoebic dysentery*: The Koya calls it *Utgary* whereas the Saora call it as *Danboridungte*. It is believed that the disease is caused by inappropriate food, over eating of chillies, excessive summer heat and by starvation also. The shaman prescribes the root of *patalagaruda (Raulphea radeshng)* along with honey for the patient to take it thrice daily.
9. *Blood Dysentery*: The Koyas call it as *Neturdak* while among the Saoras it is known as *Rangboridunote*. In both the communities it is believed that the spirit intrusion by sorcery is the cause for this disease. The Shaman among the Koya prescribes an elixir which is prepared by boiling the barks of *Tentuli (Tamarindus indica)*, *Mahula* tree (*Bassia latifolia)*, *Jammu (Syzycium integrifolia lumini)*, and *Piasala (Sptercerpus falerica)* to be taken thrice a day by the patient. The Saora *Reggmmer* prescribes an emulsion to be prepared out of *Khadira (Accasia indica)* and *Kendu (Drospyres melanoxylon)* to be taken twice by the patient.
10. *Jaundice*: The Koya call it as *Kil* and the Saora, *Rogarmeena*. This also is believed to be caused by spirit-intrusion. The Koya Shaman prescribes soaked water of *Amla (Embelica myrobalm)*, *Bahada (Terminalia balerica)* and *Horrida (Terminalia chebula)* to be taken twice daily for thirty days and the Saora shaman prescribes ground patikabellam *(Annona reticulate)* seeds, dissolved in water to be taken once daily on empty stomach with a quantity not more than four to five tea spoons at a time.
11. *Piles*: Koyas call it *Pega* and the Saoras, *Kinsum*. This also is considered by both as spirit-caused. The shaman prescribes a finger ring made of the scale of *Bajrajkapta* (a scaly ant-eater reptile).
12. *Diabetes*: The Koya call it *Wadabatita* and this is believed to be due to the displeasure of gods and goddesses. Both the Koyas and Saoras maintain that this is an incurable disease. The Koya Wadde prescribes *Jammu Cheli Rasa* (juice of *Syzycium integrifolialumini)* bark to be taken twice a day whereas the Saora *Regammar* advises the juice of *Thalkuni* leaves, an *orchid (Contella asiatica)* and ground *Methi (fenugreek)* two to three times a day.

13. *Discharge of blood with urine*: Koyas call it as *Sakabatita* and is caused by the displeasure of the supernatural. But the Saora maintain that this is caused by the consumption of the tube-well water. The Koya shaman prescribes *Saparkachu (colacasia)* and sugar cane juice whereas the Saora Regammar advises to take *Thalkunti (contella asiatica)* juice and *Jamblia juice (Citrus aurantum)* thrice a day.
14. *Goiter*: The Saora call it *Kingkingbongada* and the Koyas, *medakaya* and is believed due to supernatural wrath. Koyas prescribe a paste of *Bajramuli, Nardia, and Mustumir* to be applied over the swollen parts. The saora *Regammar* advises the juice of the roots of Bakula tree (*Mimusopa elongi)* and *Patalagaruda* plant two or three times a day.
15. *Rheumatoid Arthritis*: The Koyas call this *Peettand* and the Saoras, *Labla* and is believed to have been caused by excessive manual labour. The Shaman among them prescribes a paste made of the barks of Neem (*Aazadirachta indica)* tree, *Karanja (Carisea carandus)* tree and seeds of Datura to be applied to the affected joints. In addition half-baked *Arakha* leaves to be pasted over the joints for immediate relief.
16. *Hysteria*: The Koyas call it as *Kundel* and the Saoras, *Disung* and is believed due to spirit-intrusion. The only remedy is the exorcism of the spirit and the propitiation of the supreme god and goddess.
17. *Syphilis and Gonorrhoea*: The Koyas call it *Bakada* and the Saora, *Lablansung* and is caused according to their belief, due to the displeasure of the supernatural although they are aware that it is a sexually transmitted disease. Besides appeasing the gods and goddesses the Koya *Rotowadde* prescribes the juice of *Baruna (Cretera religiosa)* tree bark and *Dimiri (Ficus clomerata)* tree bark mixed with pulverized *Sunthi (Ginger* dehydrate) and powdered *Pipali (Piper logum*) twice a day in small quantity. The Saora Reggammar prescribes extraction of soaked *Horida (Terminalis chebula), Bahada (terminalia balerica)* and *Anala (Embelica myrobalan)* twice a day applying neem oil all over the sores.
18. *Tuberculosis*: Saora call this *Lablab* and the Koya, *Usbadogg* and is believed to be due to spirit-intrusion. Among the

Saora the *Kudunboi* propitiates *Ketumsum* on behalf of the patient. The Saora *Reggammar* prescribes powdered mixture of *Haladi (Caruma domestica), Bahada (Terminalia balerica)* and *Horida (Terminalia chebula*) twice daily. The Koya *Rotowadde* prescribes a mixture of *Asoka (Araca indica)* bark, *Aparajeeta (Cliteria ternatia)* and *Jaitri (Myristica fragram)* three times daily.

19. *Leprosy*: The Saora call it *Lablan* and the Koya, *Masa*. They attribute it to the extreme wrath of the supernatural. They believe it as incurable and the patient is excommunicated who becomes a wandering mendicant and never readmitted into the society. Such is the stigma attached to this disease that is most dreaded among them.
20. *Smallpox*: Among the Koya it is known as *Amma Tallur* and the Saora call it as *Singyol*. The Saora believe that it is caused by the anger of the goddess Matamundem and there is no treatment for this disease. The whole village worships the deity through their shaman and the priest and during evenings resin smoke is created to please the deity to contain the spread of this dreaded epidemic. Neem leaves are spread around the bed of the patient.
21. *Malaria*: It is called *Yanangbasum* by the Saora and *Wasa-edek* by the Koya. The Koya believe that it caused by witch-craft but the Saora believe it due to the intrusion of a spirit called *Yanangbasum*.The *Koya Wadde* nullifies the influence of witchcraft on the patient and among the Saora the Kudanboi or shaman blows out the influence of the spirit through magico-religious rite. The Saora *Reggammar* prepares a therapeutic powder out of Bahada *(Terminalia balerica)*, Pippala bark *(Ficus religiosa)* and Kendu seeds *(Azadir achta indica)*, for the patient to it thrice a day. The Koya Shaman prepares the medicine out of *neem* leaves, seeds, *Pippali (Piper longum)* and administers the same to the patient twice daily.
22. *Typhoid*: Among the Saora it is known as *Kaharanaghu* and among the Koya it is *Bechata-Edek*. The belief among both of them is that it is caused due to witchcraft or sorcery. The Saora worship *Durisum* and the Koya *Deudu* by their respective priests. The Koya *Wadde* prescribes a medicine made of *Garaga (Coix lachry majoba)* whereas the Saora

reggammar prescribes a medicine made of *neem* seeds, *tulasi* seeds and lemon seeds twice a day.

23. *Scabies*: The Koya call it *Dulbanga* and the Saora, *Gaji.* Children mostly contract this which is believed to be contagious among them. The Saora *Reggammar* makes a paste of *neem* leaves, *turmeric root* and *karanja* oil for application over the scabies. The Koya shaman prepares a thick solution out of these three sources.
24. *Measles*: The Saora call it *Jereing* and the Koya, *Pundku.* This is a child-disease and they believe that the malevolent spirits are responsible for this. The disease subsides if the spirit is appeased with the sacrifice of a black cock.
25. *Ringworm*: The Saora call it as *Banal* and the Koya, *Gatidula.* The disease is attributed by them to the environmental factors. The herbal medicine used for scabies also is used for this besides *Kochila* oil as an external balm.

VII
Summary and Conclusion

The tribes inhabiting the Eastern Ghats of Andhra Pradesh viz., Jatapu, Savara, Gadaba, Konda Reddy, Porja, Bagata, Khond, Konda Dora, Valmiki, Konda Kammara, Koya and Sugali were covered in this study. Most of the villages studied were on the hill top with the typical Eastern Ghats tribals in Andhra Pradesh. The size of the tribal villages studied varies within a range of 16 to 56 households, the smallest being Melikavalasa in Vizianagaram district inhabited by the Jatapu tribe and the largest being Vanjara in West Godavari District inhabited by the Konda Reddy and Sugali tribes. The population size falls within a range of 55 and 280 corresponding to the household range. The females outnumber males in the population composition in half of the villages especially in case of Jatapus and Koya.

With reference to the educational and economic status, including their occupations and landholdings, there are more number of illiterates among them than the literates with the exception of Modapali in Visakhapatnam District which is inhabited by Bagatas; Vanjara in West Godavari District which is inhabited by Konda Reddy and Sugali; and I. Polavaram which is inhabited by Konda Reddy and Konda Kammara. It may be noted that their literacy levels are also very basic as large majority of them attend/attended only the elementary school. With regard to their occupations large majority of them including women are found to be coolies with only a few of them who own land and work on their own agricultural fields including the *podu* lands. With regard to their landholding their lands are predominantly dry lands. Their annual household incomes fall within a range of Rupees 3000 to 10,700 with Dippavalasa village in Vizianagaram District inhabited by Gadaba Tribe recording highest average income while Kommu Gudem in West Godavari District inhabited by Koya Tribe recorded the lowest with an average of Rs. 3000 per annum per household.

With regard to the health status of the tribal populations covered in this study the sick in the total village population Kommugudem in West Godavari District inhabited by Koya tribe with 8 out of 88 population; Gandhinagar in Vizianagaram District inhabited by Jatapu and Konda Reddy tribes with 13 out of 80 population; and Solabam in Visakhapatnam District inhabited by Porja Tribe with 14 out of 96 population reported highest proportion of the sick in their population. Many sick cases are related to fever due to various etiologies including malaria. The sickness episodes were reported for during the last 15 days; one month, and two months; and Visakhapatnam and East Godavari Districts reported the highest number of cases during the last 15 days of this study.

This study brings out the fact that large number of tribals in these study villages are availing the services of the Primary Health Centres (PHCs). Only a few of them are still resorting to Traditional medicine mostly in Visakhapatnam District with a few cases reported from East and West Godavari Districts. The local medicine men are differently called in different districts with such names like, Yejjodu, Guru, etc, as described in Chapter IV.

The health status of the mother and the child among the tribes inhabiting the Eastern Ghats could be seen from the reproductive health of the mothers. One still birth each in Gandinagar in Vizianagaram, Injari and Doduput of Visakhapatnam District and one in Kommugudem of West Godavari District were reported. These still births reported were due to low birth weight and fluid accumulation in the feotus. Two abortion cases each were reported from I. Polavaram and Kindra villages in East Godavari. The pregnant women were given IFA tablets in almost all cases except two cases each in Injari and I. Polavaram villages and three cases in Doduput village of Visakhapatnam district. In all the cases during the fourth month of pregnancy invariably 100 IFA tablets were distributed.

Among the methods adopted for the promotion of contraceptives use, distribution of condoms and use of Copper-T and oral pills are found to be the usual methods practiced in all the PHCs with East Godavari District in the lead probably because of the high incidence of HIV/AIDS in that district. Distribution of condoms by the PHCs is found in all the PHCs of all the districts but the distribution of IEC material and advices related to spacing methods are found to be given not much importance in all the PHCs except in two or three districts (East and West Godavari and Visakhapatnam districts) reflecting the poor performance of the PHCs staff in this area. Obstructed labour and hypertensive disorders are predominant of all the maternal illnesses reported in this study. The highest number of these cases was reported from Khammam district followed by Vizianagaram. Haemorrhage, sepsis and abortions constitute insignificant proportion. Anti-natal check-ups are done by all the PHCs in all the districts both at home and in the PHCs as per the data but the authenticity of it is doubtful. However, these figures could be taken as indicative of the PHCs awareness to such a performance. Deliveries were done in the PHCs in all the districts within a range of 48-1500 per annum with Visakhapatnam leading the figures because of the high concentration of tribals (more than 14% of the population). Other obstetric services provided are the provision of 24 hours delivery services, post-natal care for mothers and the new born. Details related to the injections that were used and the interventions to save the mother and child were not provided by any of the PHCs. A few deliveries conducted by untrained persons were reported from the PHCs of Visakhapatnam and East Godavari Districts.

Emergency obstetric care and safe abortion facilities ensure the survival and health of the mother and the child. It may be noted here that some of the major initiative in Reproductive Child Health II include provision of essential obstetric services such as provision of 24 hours delivery services at all CHCs and select PHCs; post-natal care for the mother and the new born; skilled attendance at birth; emergency obstetric care at first referral units; and provision of safe abortion facilities.

In almost all the PHCs studied in all the districts referral services are found to be available except in the case of one PHC in Visakhapatnam, two in West Godavari, three in East Godavari and five in Khammam District. But in large majority of First Referral

Units (FRUs) blood storage facility is absent. It is also found that in many cases the doctors who man these PHCs do not have training in life-saving anesthetic skills, emergency obstetric management care. Although abortions are done under medical supervision there is almost an equal number of the PHCs without adequate medical supervision. Provision of quality manual vacuum aspiration facility is absent in all the PHCs except in case of two PHCs in Vizianagaram and one each in Nalgonda and Cuddapah Districts.

Auxiliary Nursing Maids (ANMs) home visits were reported in the positive by all the pregnant mothers in all the villages studied except in two cases from I. Polavaram and one each in Kommugudema and Vanjara villages. Accordingly all the women reported to have gone to their respective PHCs to avail the facilities and counselling by the ANMs and other health workers. Access to the facilities of the institutional arrangements in the PHCs is available to all the tribal villagers in all the districts studied. However, only in few cases the traditional *vaid* attended the problems related to pregnant women.

The place of delivery in most cases was either the hospital/PHC or home and a large number of them were reported to have taken place in the hospitals/PHCs. In large majority of the cases the medical doctor conducted the deliveries. In few other cases the deliveries were conducted by the health workers and the ANMs. The deliveries were reported to be normal in all the cases except in one case in Kommugudem where there was a still birth due to accumulation of fluid. None of them reported to have used contraceptives.

Ever since the Family Planning Programmes were introduced in 1952, India has progressed remarkably in areas related to maternal and child health. For example, according to the 2005 National Family Health Survey, total fertility rate is brought down from 6 to 2.9; Maternal mortality ratio to 301; infant mortality rate from 146 to 58; child mortality rate (0-4) from 57.3 to 17. However, the situation related to tribals in this area still needs to be improved.

The infant mortality rate (IMR) in 2005 is 58 per 1,000 live births (SRS, RGI Office). It is lower in urban areas at 40/1,000 live births than in rural areas which is 64/1,000 live births. Although accurate information on tribals is not available it is the highest our country has ever recorded. High IMRs are reported from the three north coastal Andhra districts of Srikakulam, Vizianagaram and Visakhapatnam Districts. The causes were attributed to poor hygienic conditions at the PHCs, low birth weight and malnutrition. Diarrhoea is the major cause and the highest number of cases were reported from Khammam District followed by Vizianagaram and Nellore Districts. Water contamination and insufficient availability of potable water in these areas could be the reasons for such high incidence. Malaria accounts for another major cause that contributes to child morbidities although there were not many mortalities. Vizianagaram, Khammam and Nellore districts registered more malaria cases. The overall neonatal deaths were very small in number and the few cases reported were due to pre-mature deliveries and sepsis.

Jhansi (2009) reports that the infant mortality rate (IMR) in the village Badbel has shown the highest IMR i.e. 428 per 1000 live births followed by Banduguda (231). Apparently, the observed high IMR among the Bondo could be due to non-representation of the entire population (Sinha, U.P—personal communication). Infant deaths take place due to a variety of factors, such as, deaths due to vaccination, preventable diseases, obstetrical complications, influence of folk beliefs and practices pertaining to the care of pregnant women, child rearing and weaning practices, general poor health of expectant mothers, undernourishment and unsafe deliveries under unhygienic conditions conducted by untrained birth attendants etc. Health facilities like immunization, TT (Tetanus) precaution, antenatal check-up, supply of IFA (Iron Folic Acid) tablets, health check-ups of the pregnant mothers are very irregular in Badbel due to its physical inaccessibility. Banduguda is only ¼ km away from Panchayat Headquarters of Mudulipada. The village is well connected by a jeepable road with Mudulipada. Presence of Anganwadi worker, Traditional Birth attendant and the performance of ANM and male health worker could be the major causes of lower IMR in Banduguda than in Badbel.

Imparting of health education to improve the general immunity of the mother and the child were the measures taken by the PHCs to promote the breast feeding of the child by the mothers. More nutritious food in addition to health education were some of the measures taken by the ICDS to promote complementary feeding.

In case of neo-natal mortality, Integrated Management of Neo-natal and Childhood Illnesses (IMNCI) was the major initiative under the Reproductive Child Health programme. This strategy includes a range of interventions to prevent and manage five major childhood illnesses such as ARI, diarrhoea, measles, malaria, and malnutrition. The major components of this strategy include, the strengthening the skills of health care workers, strengthening the health care infrastructure and the involvement of the community. It is interesting to notice that all the PHCs reported undertaking of the strengthening of skills of their health care workers. The involvement of the community, which is very crucial to improve the health standards of the people, was reported in all the PHCs except in Srikakulam District where four PHCs reported in the negative. In case of Anti-malarial programmes too the district reported in the negative. Home-based neo-natal care was reported from all the PHCs except three in Vizianagaram and two in Visakhapatnam. The training of the ANMs is a mixed bag as large number of them, 20 from Srikakulam and 10 from Vizianagaram Districts reported in the negative. In other districts a small number of them reported positively.

The National Health Policy (1983) accorded high priority to the immunization of children, and universal immunization against the six vaccine preventable diseases (VPD). All the PHCs studied have administered the vaccinations for polio, diphtheria, pertussis, measles and tuberculosis. The pregnant women invariably were given Tetanus toxoid injections and the babies between 12 and 23 months old were administered vaccines.

Immunizations given to the children of the villages and the neo-natal care given by the PHCs agree with the data collected from the health personnel of the PHCs. After the delivery the umbilical cord was invariably cut by a blade and it, therefore, seems to be the usual practice among all the tribals in these districts. In all these villages the vaccinations to the infants are given for polio, diphtheria, pertussis, tetanus, measles and tuberculosis. In almost all the villages, home-based neo-natal care was given by the PHCs except in two cases of Injari and three cases in Doduput villages of Visakhapatnam District. All the tribals of all the villages studied own health cards which indicate the dates on which vaccinations were given to the children. The pregnant women of these tribal villages were all given tetanus toxoid injections during their antenatal period. But hepatitis B and injectable Vi antigen were not at all given. The children between ages 12 and 23 months received vaccinations for BCG, polio3, DPT3, measles, and all other vaccines. The children between the ages of 12 to 23 months received all the primary vaccines. Ulipirivalasa of Srikakulam District and Dippavalasa of Vizianagaram District recorded the highest number of vaccinations given for polio during the last year. Administration of Polio vaccine seems to be very successful in all the PHCs.

Mid day meal scheme—the national programme of nutritional support to primary education was launched on 15th August, 1995 to give a boost to universal primary education.

Nutritional status of the tribals from the Anganwadi centres point out a very large number of cases related to anaemia in all the districts. Women between the ages 15 to 49 and babies between the ages of 6 to 36 months were found to be anaemic in large number. The National Goitre Control programme is in operation in only Srikakulam, Vizianagaram and Mahboobnagar Districts with the other districts reporting in the negative. In fact a very large number of Goitre cases were reported from Visakhapatnam district three/four decades ago due to iodine deficiency. Iodized salt supply was reported in all the PHCs of all the districts except in West Godavari and Khammam. A few Vitamin deficiency disorders were reported especially for bitot spots and softening of cornea.

In all the AWCs nutritious supplements such as *dal*, oil and rice are being provided. In addition, services like periodic health check-ups, immunizations, growth promoting supplementary feeding, referral services, early childhood care and pre-school education and distribution of nutrition supplements to promote child health are being provided. Only in a few place periodic health check-ups and immunizations are not regularly done as found in the AWCs of Cuddapah, Visakhapatnam and Mahboobnagar districts. It may be noted here that apart from the distribution of nutrition supplements, the AWC is the hub for the delivery of primary health care interventions by the ANM such as immunization, distribution of Iron Folic Acid and Vitamin-A supplements, distribution of oral contraceptive pills, growth monitoring and promotion and health education and counselling to mothers.

Children between the ages of 6 to 35 months were found anaemic in all the villages studied. Although the data were in single digits in all the villages, anaemia seems to be the major cause for children's morbidity in all the villages studied. Same is the case with women belonging to 15 to 49 years of age as many of them were found to be anaemic in this study. Thus anaemia emerges to be the leading cause for the morbidity among both the mothers and the children of these tribal villages. The Goitre control programme was not in operation in any of these villages studied although the PHC data reported it to be in operation in three districts as mentioned earlier. Only one case each of Goitre was reported from Ulipirivalasa of Srikakulam District, Dippavalasain Vizianagaram district and Modapali in Visakhapatnam District. Iodized salt also was not distributed in these villages. Only one case of Vitamin-A deficiency which caused corneal ulcers was reported from Gandhinagar in Vizianagaram District.

The performance of the ICDS as reported by the villagers was satisfactory. The tribals of the villages studied reported that the ICDS functioning in providing immunizations and antenatal care was satisfactory except in case of 20 villagers in Ulipirivalasa in Srikakulam District and 16 in Dippavalasa of Vizianagaram District. All the tribals reported that they were having regular health check-ups except 28 in Ulipirivalasa, 26 in Rangapuram, both from Srikakulam District, 19 from Gandhinagar and 28 in Dippavalasa in Vizianagaram District.

With reference to growth promotion of the children and supplementary feeding the answer was negative invariably in all the villages. The availability of referral services received responses from only 6 villages with three of them answering in the positive and other three in the negative. With regard to the early childhood care of the pre-school children the tribals in all the villages except in Gandhinagar of Vizianagaram answered in the positive but the adolescent girls were not given any health education including nutrition. But in case of the pregnant women such health education seems to have been imparted except in case of Gandhinagar. The nursing mothers too received such an education except again in case of Gandhinagar. Mothers seem to have been given orientation in using ORS solution. With regard to the treatment of common diseases and injuries all the PHCs reported that ORS packets are available with them. The ORS meant for mothers also is available in all the PHCs except 2 in Visakhapatnam, 3 in East Godavari and 1 in West Godavari. In addition to ORS, Zinc tablets are also supplied except in 2 PHCs in Visakhapatnam and 6 in East

Godavari district. ASHA is found to be active in all the villages under the PHCs studied except in Visakhapatnam and East Godavari Districts.

The ICDSs in all the Districts reported working for NNAP Programme. The National Vit-A programme is not in operation in any of the villages. The tribals perceive the role of ASHA is to distribute tablets, imparting health education and rendering assistance to the ANMs. The medical personnel assert that the role of ASHA as distribution of tablets for common illnesses like cough, cold and fever, rendering assistance to the ANMS, and imparting health education to the villagers, etc. Except in Doduput village in Visakhapatnam in all the other villages there is the presence of ASHA. Although a few of the villagers answered in the negative it has to be considered as their ignorance of such a person ASHA. Janani Suraksha Yojna scheme has identified the critical role of ASHA in facilitating delivery by a poor pregnant female and arranging for referral transport. With regard to the performance of ASHA large majority of the tribal villagers expressed satisfaction. Only, a few of them answered in the negative. With regard to ASHAs training in dealing with the generic diseases the responses invariably were in the negative.

The National Nutritional Anaemia Prophylaxis Programme (NNAP) is in operation in all the PHCs in all the districts except in 7 PHCs of Visakhapatnam District and 9 in East Godavari District. In all the PHCs studied, IFA (Iron and Folic Acid) tablets are being distributed to the pregnant women. The blindness prevention programme is in operation in all the PHCs except in 9 PHCs in Visakhapatnam district. A large number of TB cases were reported from Vizianagaram and Srikakulam Districts and the causative factors were found to be the habit of smoking, the types of foods they consume and living in crowded and congested rooms.

"Available evidence suggests that poverty is the prime cause for ill health, persistent morbidity and early death. However, lack of access to right foods: iron, protein and micro-nutrients such as iodine and vitamins, is the principal cause for the very high incidence of nutritional deficiency diseases: anaemia, radesh, night blindness, goitre, etc. These factors combined with lack of access to basic health care services is the main reason for the unexceptionally adverse differentials with the more developed parts of the State: maternal mortality is eight per 1,000, (going up to 25 among some tribal groups) as against 4 per 1,000 for the State; infant mortality rate is 120-150 per 1000 compared to 72 per 1,000; and while it is 9 per 1,000 crude death rate, with 30 per cent under-five mortality for the State, among some of the major tribal groups such as Savaras, Gadabas and Jatapus, the death rate is as high as 15-20 per 1,000 with over 50 per cent of deaths of children under five" (Sujatha Rao,1998: 481).

"Lack of accommodation, poor infrastructure, large-scale absenteeism and vacancies, poorly trained and unmotivated manpower, are thus the reasons for the near absence of health care services (page 482)".

"(in case of) TB and malaria, the tribals suffer disproportionately to their population—the rate of incidence of TB among tribals is estimated to be double and under malaria, case incidence is estimated to be over 18 per 1,000, mostly of P Falciparum variety, accounting for 75 per cent of the State's total deaths on account of malaria......Despite evidence of the adverse impact malaria has in exacerbating anaemia, or, in finding that 20 per cent of mortality of women in the productive age group is due to TB, the implementation of these programmes have not been incorporated" (Sujatha Rao,1998: 481).

In view of the strong association of TB, malaria, AIDS, STD to reproductive health, the policy framework falls short in not assessing the operational inadequacies for improving the programme implementation of these public health programmes—for example, data shows that most malarial deaths are on account of delayed treatment. The average time taken in tribal areas for a blood slide to be examined and results informed is six weeks to six months. On account of inadequate budgets for travel allowances, workers tend to wait for 10-15 days till enough number of slides are collected before handling them in for testing and some of the slides get spoiled in that process. As malaria is endemic all over India, the National Malaria Control Programme (NMCP) emphasizes the indoor residual spraying of DDT. All the PHCs in all the districts have reported the use of DDT spraying in their jurisdiction.

The diarrhoeal episodes are very common among the tribals and the etiology could be traced to consumption of contaminated water. The water shortages in many of the areas and the quality of even bore-well water, their age-old cultural practices usually compound this situation further. Imparting health education, to drink water only after boiling and cooling, plays a very important role in containing the diarrhoeal episodes. In our study, the highest number of such cases was reported from Visakhapatnam, East Godavari, West Godavari and Nellore in that order. As per the diarrhoeal deaths reported from the PHCs a few such cases were reported from Visakhapatnam (4), East Godavari (6), and West Godavari (2). In all the PHCs, administration of ORS solution to prevent dehydration was reported.

Dots coverage refers to the number of cases covered under DOTS (Directly Observed Treatment-Short Course) under the revised National Tuberculosis Control Programme (RNTCP). East Godavari, Khammam, Nellore, Vizianagaram and West Godavari reported the highest coverage under DOTS. A very high number of vector borne diseases were reported from Visakhapatnam and East Godavari Districts.

One of the essential components of the Primary Health Care approach is the appropriate treatment of common illnesses and injuries at the peripheral level. An ANM manning the sub-centre is provided with prophylactic Kit A and essential drugs Kit B to manage such common illnesses. ARIs (acute respiratory infections) and diarrhoea are the two leading causes of childhood morbidity and mortality. Kit A contains IFA (large and small), Vitamin A solution, cotrimoxazole tablets, ORS packets, disposable delivery kit; Kit B contains methyl ergometrine maleate tablets/injection, paracetamol tablets, mebendazole, dicyclomine tablets, chloamphenicol eye ointment, povidone Iodine, cetrimide powder, cotton and bandages. All the ANMs in the study area have reported positively about carrying of these kits in all the PHCs in all the districts.

To prevent and control locally endemic diseases DDT spraying within the house and surroundings of the house was undertaken in all the study villages in all the districts. All the cases of locally endemic diseases reported were diarrhoeal cases and fevers caused mostly due to malaria. The preventive and control measures taken relate to keeping the houses and surroundings clean and neat. Health education again plays an important role in this context too. Many of the respondents expressed their ignorance as to the measures initiated at the village level in this regard.

With regard to the treatment of common illnesses and injuries large majority of the tribals in all the study villages in all the districts are availing treatment at the PHCs with a few exception of 9 in Rangapuram in Srikakulam District, 8 in Dippavalasa of Vizianagaram District, 6 in Modapali, 8 in Doduput, and 9 in Downuru in Visakhapatnam District, 7 in Kindra of East Godavari District, and 4 in Kommugudem of West Godavari District who reported to be still using the services of the local traditional healers. Of course, the PHC Doctor is mostly preferred by all the tribals in all the villages A few of them, 9 from Rangapuram, 8 from Dippavalasa, 6 from Solabam, 8 from Injari, 9 from Doduput, 7 from Kindra and 4 from Kommugudem preferred ANMs. This preference of ANMs is mostly due to the long absence of the Doctor from the PHC. As in many PHCs it is observed that the Doctors go on a long leave making the posts lying vacant for a long time. A little more dedication and responsibility is found wanting according to many tribal respondents in addition to have more health education from her. There is no such thing as school sanitation in all the villages studied except in Modapali and Doduput in Visakhapatnam District in Kindra and Vanjara of East and West Godavari districts respectively.

The Integrated Management of Neonatal and Childhood Illnesses (IMNCI) is followed in all the PHCs studied except in case of 11 PHCs in Visakhapatnam and 5 in East Godavari districts. The syndrome based diagnosis is practiced by all the health workers in all the PHCs except in Visakhapatnam and a few in East Godavari (4), and West Godavari (3). Kits for sexually Transmitted Infections (STI) are in good supply in all the PHCs except in Srikakulam district. All the PHCs have reported that the drugs are available on a regular basis in their centres. The list of essential drugs required is incomplete with only PHCs in Srikakulam district providing relevant information which reflects on the ignorance of the PHC staff as to what we mean by 'essential drugs'. In fact the kits A and B contain most of the essential drugs and all the Sub-Centres of the PHCs of this study are being supplied with the kits containing essential drugs every six months. As to the availability of standard treatment guidelines it was answered in the positive by all the PHCs except one in Srikakulam District, two in Vizianagaram and four in Visakhapatnam PHCs. With regard to the in-service training of the PHC staff except in case of 7 PHCs in Visakhapatnam, 8 in East Godavari, 2 in West Godavari districts, all other PHCs reported in the positive.

With regard to water and sanitation no technological improvisations were introduced in all the study villages but IEC (information, education and communication) campaigns were undertaken in all these villages. The paramedical staff of the PHCs maintains that they are attending to the problems related to the sanitation within the villages with the exception of 2 PHCs in Vizianagaram District. They are in the practice of imparting health education to the villagers with the exception of 5 PHCs in Visakhapatnam District. In an earlier study (Rao, R.S, 2007) it was pointed out that the health aspect covered under IEC campaigns are about polio, water sanitation, HIV/AIDS, environmental sanitation, nutritious, diet, fevers, antenatal care, mother and child health, diarrhoea, mothers milk and mosquito nets. Of all the messages, the information pertaining to polio, HIV/AIDS, environmental sanitation and fevers attracted the community to a large extent. Most often the tribals were provided with written information which may not suit the illiterate tribal population. Therefore, the tribals felt that charts with bigger illustrations along with explanation by the health care providers would be more appropriate in this regard. Periodic meetings, stage shows and *kala jatharas* (fairs) may be more effective. Rallies with school children on health related aspects at road side villages are also more effective in sensitizing the people.

When the question of their awareness of the essential drugs devised by Indian Public Health standards they all have invariably replied in the positive. With reference to their knowledge related to the protocols for diarrhoea and immunization schedules they all have replied in the positive. It is only in case of TB, 8 PHCs and in case of leprosy 11 PHCs all in Visakhapatnam replied in the negative.

With regard to any one trying to bring about any behavioural changes among them the reply was in negative by all the tribals of this study. As to their awareness of Nirmal Gram Puraskar the answer mostly was in the negative except in case of 30 tribals in Modapali, 20 in Doduput in Visakhapatnam district, 20 in I. Polavaram and 39 in Kindra of East Godavari Districts and 56 in Vanjara of West Godavari District. With regard to their personal hygiene related to cleaning of teeth, about one-fourth of the households reported once in three days and another one-fourth once in two days. Only half of them reported it as once everyday. Vanjara in East Godavari, Ulipirivalasa in Srikakulam District, I.

Polavaram and Kindra in East Godavari Districts reported large number of tribals cleaning their teeth once in three days.

With regard to how often they change clothes about half of them reported it as once in three days and the remaining half once in five days. This partly reflects on their economic status. Large majority of them were found to be washing their clothes in the stream water and the rest of them using the well water or hand pump. The major sources of potable water for these tribals are the open well, the bore well and the stream. In the study villages still 40 per cent of them are using stream for their drinking purpose. As water borne diseases among the tribals constitute highest proportion their etiology could be traced to such a practice of consuming the stream water. Boiling of the water before drinking was reported in the negative by all the tribals. Of course, boiling requires more firewood which could be another problem for most of the tribals. About 36 per cent tribal households reported not using soap to wash their bodies probably again due to their poverty.

A large majority of the tribals are found to be using fire-wood for cooking purpose. Only a few of them are using cooking gas and majority of them are from West Godavari District, 22 households (100%) from Kommugudem and 16 are from Vanjara. The rest are from Kindra from East Godavari, Downuru and Modapali from Visakhapatnam district. The food is reported to have been undercooked many a time which could be one of the causes for their ill health. In all the villages defecation is done in the open places on the road side as access to toilets is almost negligible with a few exceptions of using the latrines as in case of 20 in Vanjira, 15 in Kindra, 10 in Dippavalasa. Washing of hands thoroughly after defecation also was reported in the negative by all the tribals. Not a single HIV/AIDS case was reported in this study sample although there are some cases reported among the tribals from other areas. All the staff of the PHCs asserted that they are engaged in the activities related to the prevention of HIV/AIDs and other life-style diseases. The IEC (Information, education and communication) activities included pasting wall posters and catchy slogans wherever possible in addition to arranging rallies periodically to create more and more awareness about these diseases. Monitoring of the impact of these activities is also undertaken by all the PHCs. Health melas are organized periodically in all the PHCs invariably.

The urban orientation of the health personnel pose problems to the functioning of the PHCs. The Health survey 2003 reports 35 per cent of the PHCs without Doctors. Large majority of the tribals expressed the need for more number of health professionals posted in their area. Many posts in many of the PHCs are found to be lying vacant. For example, in Sulha Nagar, Khammam the vacancies are as follows: Med. Officer: 1; HEO;1; OP Asst: 1; LT: 1; Night ANM: 1; Health Asst: 2; MPHS-M: 2; MPHS-F: 1; MLT: 1;Office attendant: 1;Clinical ANM: 1

Only a small number of the health staff are staying in the quarters for varied reasons. Many of them also expressed that the communication facilities in their area must be improved. During the last year, sickness was reported in all the households with 2 mortalities in Rangapuram of Srikakulam District and one in Doduput village of Visakhapatnam District. Health campaigns were reported in 5 of the villages studied and except in Modapali in no other village health *melas* were conducted. During the last month of the study, except in a few households in three villages, all the households in all the villages in all the Districts sickness was reported.

Fevers occupy the top position followed by scabies and respiratory diseases. Stagnant pools of water prove to be the breeding places for mosquitoes which cause malaria. Skin infections, mostly scabies, seem to be high among the children in the age group of 5-15 due to insufficient washing of hands and feet after play and the incidence is high in the months of February, March, April and May in which there usually is acute shortage of water. Body pains are due to carrying head loads of their daily necessities, water and firewood. Worm infestations are due to consumption of contaminated water.

Interview with the Medical Staff working in the Tribal area and the tribals yielded some useful suggestions to improve the state of things related to improve the tribal health standards. For a question how the outreach services can be improved, the Staff in the PHC in Munnanor, Mahboobnagar districts suggested appointment of a doctor in 104 and 108 ambulances. As PHCs do not have quarters for their staff many of them are staying outside their place of work. So construction of quarters is a very badly felt requirement in many places which would improve the performance of the PHCs. Conducting more and more awareness camps on AIDs would be effective in IEC campaigns. In order to promote breast feeding, counselling of couples during antenatal check up and making them to feed the baby early should be done in right earnest.

The staff of the PHC at Chitvel in Cuddapah felt that imparting health education related to family planning, puberty, personal hygiene, diet, baby care, nutrition, and pregnancies would certainly improve their health. Early registration of pregnancies is very much wanted in many cases as it would facilitate timely referrals.

The study also brought to light in Vepinapi, the Pharmacist administers medicines in the absence of the Medical Doctor who attends the PHC once in two days. It was also reported that even on the Polio Vaccination day he was not present, but only the ANMs were present. One staff nurse post is vacant here. There are also 6 male multi-purpose health workers posted at this PHC. They get Rs. 5200 p.m. but the salary is being paid once in six months and that too not in full.

In Chitvel the PHC Doctor stays still 12 noon and attends only the emergency cases. The functioning of the PHC in Railway Koduru is satisfactory but for the cleaning/sweeping of the PHC and the surroundings for which the helpers are demanding high amounts. It seems there is no provision to meet such a contingency and the Doctor posted there is finding it difficult to meet the expenditure. The Staff Nurses are reckless in treating the patients in the absence of the Doctor and indifferent to their work.

In Amarabad there is a Government Civil Hospital with three doctors and two Staff Nurses, one Pharmacist, one Water boy, two ANMs and two Thotis but the hospital is not maintained well. The Doctors are not available according to the timings.

In Balamoor the Doctor comes to the PHC once in three days. A second grade ANM is present. The Staff nurse expressed ignorance with certain aspects contained in our schedule.

The PHC Doctor in Tekulapalli is sincere to his work and disclosed that there is lot of political pressure and interference in his work. When a political leader comes he has to be shown utmost respect offering him a chair. As the Hospital has a Hospital Development fund with these political leaders as members of the committee. They do not attend the meeting in time. Even the District Medical Officer has to wait for these 'illiterate' leaders. They do not speak much in the meeting but expect the DMO to provide them food after the meeting. If he fails to do so they make a lot of nuisance. They also ask the DMO to part with some money of the fund.

In Chandrugouda, the Doctor seems to be not aware of certain things in the schedule. In this area most of them are Lambadis and a small number of them Koyas. In VR Puram 24 hours PHC; there is one staff nurse and another on contract basis who works in two shifts.

The Kusimi PHC staff in Srikakulam District opined that posting of sufficient staff, providing more budget for drugs, improvement of infra-structural facilities and availability of a vehicle for emergency transport would improve the functioning of the PHCs. According to them the inherent problems in the existing programmes include communication problems and poor transportation facility.

In general, the Anganwadis seem to be functioning satisfactorily. The teacher is 10th class qualified and according to her the ICDS provides food once in 25 days; Rice, wheat flour, *pesarapappu* (green dal), and oil are supplied; On every first Wednesday immunizations are administered to the pregnant women and to the women who already delivered babies. They also look after 5 years old education and the 2 years old children are given immunizations. To those women who already delivered, once in 25 days, 2 kgs rice, 200 gms oils, 1 kg *pesarapappu* (green dal) is given. According to the Anganawadi teacher in Golla Bajar, peanuts, jowar, *putnalu* with sugar are ground into flour which is called *pillulu* and the pregnant women are given once in 15 days, one and a half kg flour. All other centres are given the standard provisions except this one as they receive only this flour.

To sum up, the solutions to the problem areas in administering to the health needs of the tribals include :

1. Tribal needs assessment has to be done in every tribal area.
2. Integration of Traditional Health Care Practices with the Modern System.
3. Ensure tribal participation in planning and implementation of health programmes employing a bottom-up approach.
4. Appointment of doctors in 104/108 ambulatory services.
5. To construct quarters for the PHC staff to make them stay in the village.

6. To conduct more and more of Health Education camps/ melas by IEC interventions. Although the ITDAs are doing good work many of the tribals are not aware of many of the programmes beneficial to them. In this respect there are inter-tribal differences, hence health education on a war footing is warranted.
7. To check the large scale absenteeism of the doctors working in the tribal areas.
8. To fill up all the existing vacancies in the PHCs in tribal areas.
9. To provide training programmes for the Staff including the Doctors of the PHCs to update their knowledge.
10. To take necessary steps to check the political interference in the day-to-day administration of the PHCs.
11. Provision of enough funds for essential drugs and emergency services including vehicles at least for a cluster of PHCs.
12. Construction/renovation of PHC buildings and repairs to mobile medical units including improvements in infrastructure.
13. Construction of Roads to access the PHCs.
14. To take up conversion of some of the PHCs into CHCs.
15. To develop a system of accountability and better use of finances in the distribution of medicines.
16. As many of the health programmes are not reaching the interior places in the agency areas sufficient vehicles may be provided to the PHCs.
17. The PHC staff in this connection has to be sufficiently motivated, if necessary by providing some incentives.
18. IEC Interventions have to be increased by the distribution of pamphlets, charts, leaflets, booklets, wall posters, Rajiv Arogyasri camps including arranging periodic melas especially on *shandy* (tribal market) days. Exploring and propagating the concept of '*mee sneham*' (your friendship) by group meeting is one of the things in the successful interventions.
19. Encouraging the use of herbal medicine (ethno-medicine) is desirable as it is affordable and efficacious in case of some ailments.

20. Need for a new paradigm (Sujatha Rao's): The development paradigm will need to make health centre stage in the over all development strategy.
21. To create a separate category of 'All India Tribal Health Services' on par with IAS for the better Tribal Health administration.
22. The Tribal Health policy has to be evolved making it 'tribal oriented' rather than "building and doctor oriented".
23. As the tribals desire charts with bigger illustrations along with explanation by the health care providers would be more appropriate in IEC exercises.
24. Periodic meetings with the tribals by the PHC staff, stage shows and *kala jatharas* (fairs are more effective in IEC Campaigns.
25. Rallies with school children on health related aspects at road side villages are also more effective in sensitizing the people.
26. Providing health insuarance coverage for all the tribals at a nominal cost.
27. There should be proper coordinationbetween all the Government Departments in improving the health status of the tribals.

APPENDIX I

List of Villages Studied

S. No.	*District*	*Villages*
1.	Visakhapatnam	Solabam
2.		Modapali
3.		Injari
4.		Doduput
5.		Downuru
6.	Srikakulam	Ulipirivalasa
7.		Rangapuram
8.	Vizianagaram	Gandhinagar
9.		Melikavalasa
10.		Dippavalasa
11.	Nelluru	
12.	Kammam	
13.	Mehabubnagar	
14.	Cuddapah	
15.	West Godavari	Kommu G.
		Vanjara
16.	East Godavari	I. Polavar
		Kindra

APPENDIX II
List of PHCs and CHCs Studied

S. No.	*District*	*Village*	*PHC/CHC*
1.	Visakhapatnam	Paderu	CHC
2.	"	Araku Valley	CHC
3.	"	Hukumpeta	PHC
4.	"	Dumbriguda	PHC
5.	"	Peadabayalu	PHC
6.	"	Munchangiputtu	PHC
7.	"	G. Madugula	PHC
8.	"	Lothugadda	PHC
9.	"	Anathagiri	PHC
10.	"	G.K. Veedi	PHC
11.	"	Koyyuru	PHC
12.	Srikakulam	Kusimi	PHC
13.	"	Bhamini	PHC
14.	"	Donubai	PHC
15.	"	Marripadu	PHC
16.	"	Doliseela	PHC
17.	Vizianagaram	K.R.B. Puram	CHC
18.	"	Kurupam	PHC
19.	"	Kumarada	PHC
20.	Nelluru	Kunavaram	PHC
21.	"	Napinopi	PHC
22.	"	Rebhapalli	PHC
23.	Khammam	Julurpad	PHC
24.	"	Chandrugonda	PHC
25.	"	Subhanagar	PHC
26.	"	Tulasipaka	PHC
27.	"	Charla	PHC
28.	Mehboobnagar	Amrabad	PHC
29.	"	Munnanur	PHC
30.	Cuddapah	Chitvel	PHC
31.	West Godavari	P.R. Gudem	CHC
32.	"	Jeelugumilli	PHC
33.	"	Kondrukota	PHC

(*Cont.*)

(*Cont.*)

S. No.	*District*	*Village*	*PHC/CHC*
34.	West Godavari	Buttaigudem	PHC
35.	"	Vinjaram	PHC
36.	"	K.R. Puram	PHC
37.	East Godavari	Gangavaram	PHC
38.	"	Yellavaram	PHC
39.	"	Rajaommangi	PHC
40.	"	Devipatnam	PHC
41.	"	Jaddangi	PHC
42.	"	Pidatamamidi	PHC
43.	"	Indukuripeta	CHC
44.	"	P. Gadda	PHC
45.	"	Maredumilli	PHC
46.	"	Narasapuram	PHC
47.	"	Chavitidibbalu	PHC
48.	"	Duppulapalem	PHC
49.	"	Boduluru	PHC

APPENDIX III
Tribal Health in Eastern Ghats

(PROJECT SPONSORED BY THE MINISTRY OF TRIBAL AFFAIRS, GOVERNMENT OF INDIA)

Name of the Village : Tribe : Mandal : District :
Name of the Respondent : Sex : Age :

Household Schedule

S. No.	*Name of the Member Starting with HH*	*Relation-ship to HH*	*Sex M/F*	*Age*	*Marital Status (M, UM, D, W)*	*Education*	*Occupation*		*Landholding (in acres)*		*Average Monthly Income*
							Primary	*Secondary*	*Wet*	*Dry*	

In your observation :

(a) How many of them are looking healthy; (b) How many are sick; (c) Are there any sick in the family now; (d) If so, record the sickness; (e) Since how long; (f) Treatment from whom; (g) Why such a preference; (h) Is there any difficulty in getting treatment; (i) Any other relevant observation related to their health.

(*Appendix III—Contd.*)

Mother and Child Health (Ask the Mother)

(Take the help of ASHA/ANM/Local Health Worker to fill the Schedule)

1. Total Number of Conceptions: Live births: Still births: Abortions:
2. Reasons for child death, if any:
3. Were you given IFA tablets during pregnancy: Yes/No
4. If yes, how many:— in what month:
5. Did the ANM visit you at home during last pregnancy: Yes/No
6. If yes, did you visit the health facility: Yes/No
7. If yes, where did you go: (a) Traditional *vaid;* (b) PHC; (c) ANM/Health Worker; (d) Others
8. If No, why:
9. Were you advised to go to PHC for delivery:
10. Where did the delivery/deliveries take place:
11. Who conducted the delivery:
12. Was the delivery normal: Yes/No
13. If no, give details:
14. Do you use contraceptives: Yes/No
    If yes, what kind: supplied by: How often used:
15. Object used to cut the umbilical cord:
16. Home-based neo-natal care given by PHC/Sub-Centre: given/not given

Immunization

17. Do you have card indicating vaccinations given: Yes/No
18. Are the vaccinations to infants given for—
    (a) Polio: Yes/No;
    (b) Diphtheria: Yes/No;
    (c) Pertussis: Yes/No;
    (d) Tetanus: Yes/No;
    (e) Measles: Yes/No;
    (f) Tuberculosis: Yes/No.
19. If vaccinations are not given, give the reasons:
20. Are the pregnant women given these during antenatal period:
    (a) Tetanus Toxoid Vaccination: Yes/No;

(*Appendix III—Contd.*)

(b) Hepatitis B vaccine: Yes/No

(c) Injectable Vi antigen Typhoid vaccine: Yes/No

21. The children aged 12-23 months received:
    (a) all primary vaccinations: Yes/No
    (b) Measles vaccination by the age of one year: Yes/No
22. How many children received Polio vaccine last year during Pulse polio campaigns?
23. How many children aged 12-23 months received the vaccination for the following:
    BCG: Polio3: DPT3: Measles: All Vaccines:
24. How many did not receive and why:

Nutrition

25. How many children of 6-35 months are found anaemic?
26. How many married women in the age group 15-49 who are found anaemic?
27. Is the Indian National Goitre Control Programme (NGCP) in operation?
28. How many cases of goitre are reported (due to iodine deficiency)?
29. Is iodized salt in supply in your village? Yes/No
30. If yes, who supplies?
31. How many Vitamin A Deficiency Disorders are reported (VAD) (a) corneal ulcers: (b) softening of cornea (keratomalacia): (c) Bitot spots:

Performance of ICDS (ask the ICDS in-charge officer)

32. What nutrition supplements are provided?
33. Describe the functioning of the Anganwadi centre with reference to the following:
    (a) in the delivery of primary health care interventions by the ANM such as immunization;
    (b) distribution of Iron Folic Acid and Vitamin A supplements;
    (c) distribution of oral contraceptive pills and other contraceptives;
    (d) growth monitoring and promotion; and
    (e) health education and counselling to mothers.

(Appendix III—Contd.)

34. Describe the Mid-Day Meal Programme:
35. Do the centres serve as immunization/antenatal care/ supplementary feed centres for 6 months to 2 years old children? Yes/No; If no, why:

Are these services provided for Children under	*1 year*	*1-3 years*	*3-6 years*
36. Health check-ups	Yes/No	Yes/No	Yes/No
37. Immunizations	Yes/No	Yes/No	Yes/No
38. Growth Promotion and Supplementary Feeding	Yes/No	Yes/No	Yes/No
39. Referral Services	Yes/No	Yes/No	Yes/No
40. Early Childhood Care and Pre-school Education	Yes/No	Yes/No	Yes/No
Nutrition and Health education given for			
41. Adolescent Girls (11-18 years)	Yes/No	Yes/No	Yes/No
42. Pregnant Woman	Yes/No	Yes/No	Yes/No
43. Nursing Mothers	Yes/No	Yes/No	Yes/No
44. All Women (15-45 years)	Yes/No	Yes/No	Yes/No

45. Do you work for the National Nutritional Anaemia Prophylaxis Programme (NNAP)
46. Are iron and folic acid distributed for (i) pregnant women: Yes/No
    (ii) (To prevent anaemia among pregnant women and children): Yes/No
47. For how many days:
48. Do you work for National Vitamin A Prophylaxis Programme (for Prevention of Blindness in operation): Yes/No
49. Describe the role of ASHA:

Prevention and Control of Locally Endemic Diseases

50. Is there indoor residual spraying surrounding your house with DDT:
51. How many cases are reported in your family during last year for the following:
    (a) HIV/AIDS
    (b) Diarrhoeal Diseases

(*Appendix III—Contd.*)

(c) Malaria
(d) Filaria
(e) Japanese Encephalitis
(f) Dengue
(g) Chickungunya
(h) Leprosy

52. What preventive and control measures are taken for each of the above (describe):

Treatment of Common Illnesses and Injuries

53. Where do you go for treatment:
54. Who is your traditional healer:
55. By what name he is called:
56. For what ailments do you consult him:
57. How much fees does he charge:
58. Describe his method of treatment:
59. Who are the other medical practitioners available to you:
60. Who do you prefer: PHC/Traditional healer/RMP/others specify)
61. Do you have ASHA in your village:
62. What services do you receive from ASHA:
63. Are you satisfied with her performance:
64. What else do you expect from her:
65. Are the mothers oriented to prepare and use the ORS solution at home when her child has diarrhoea: Yes/No
66. The community level link worker (ASHA) got trained to deal with generic ailments at village/hamlet level: Yes/No

Water Supply and Sanitation

67. Any incentives provided for constructing individual household latrine units: Yes/No
68. If yes, what kind:
69. Is there any such thing as School Sanitation:
70. Are there any technology improvisations:
71. Is there any IEC (information, education, communication) Campaign involving Panchayati Raj Institutions, Co-operatives, Women Groups, Self Help Groups, NGOs: Yes/No

(*Appendix III—Contd.*)

72. If yes, describe the activities:
73. Has anybody tried to bring about relevant behavioural changes for improved sanitation and hygiene practices: Yes/No
74. If yes, give details:
75. Are you aware of "Nirmal Gram Puraskar" for fully sanitized and open defecation free Gram Panchayats: Yes/No

Health Education

Personal Habits

76. How often do you clean your teeth and body:
77. If so, do you use soap/paste or other things:
78. How often do you change clothes:
79. Where do you wash clothes/utensils:
80. Source of potable water:
81. Do you boil the water and drink:
82. How do you cook your food:
83. Is it well cooked/undercooked:
84. Where do you defecate:
85. Do you wash your hands thoroughly:
86. Any effective Communication made/being made for behaviour changes to prevent HIV/AIDS and other life style diseases: Yes/No
87. If yes, give details:
88. Mention the IEC Interventions in detail:
89. Explain the Role of Mass Media in promoting health in your village:
90. Specify contextual needs, if any:
91. Was there any recent health campaign conducted in your village:
92. Were there any health *melas* organized to spread health awareness:

Episodes of Sickness during Last Month/Last Year

93. Any sickness in the family during the last month: Yes/No

(*Appendix III—Contd.*)

94. If yes, give details:
95. Who diagnosed What and who gave the treatment:
96. Result:
97. Sickness during the last year:
98. Details: Treated by: Result:
99. Any mortalities during the last year: Reasons:

APPENDIX IV

Tribal Health in Eastern Ghats

*(Sponsored by Ministry of Tribal Affairs,
Government of India)*

PHC/CHC/SUB-CENTRE-SCHEDULE

1. Mother and Child Health

(If the answer is 'No' please explain why.
Answers pertain to exclusively tribals.
Data related to immediate last year)

1. What measures are adopted for the promotion of contraceptives:
2. Does the PHC/CHC/Sub-Centre supply contraceptives: Yes/No
   If yes, what kind: Supplied by:
   How often supplied:
3. During the last year how many cases are related to:
   (a) Haemorrhage
   (b) Sepsis
   (c) Abortion
   (d) Obstructed Labour
   (e) Hypertensive disorders
4. Anti-natal Check-ups during the last one year:
   (a) How many:
   (b) Where: PHC/Home
5. What are the essential Obstetric Services provided (check):
   (a) Anti-natal Care
   (b) Institutional Safe Delivery Practices
   (c) Post-natal care for early and timely detection of emergencies
   (d) Provision of 24 hours delivery services at all CHCs and PHCs
   (e) Post-natal care for mothers and new born
   (f) What kinds of injections are given (specify):
   (g) What are the interventions initiated to save the mother and child:

(h) How many institutional deliveries during the last five years:
(i) Deliveries conducted by trained personnel in Domicillary delivery
(j) Deliveries conducted by untrained personnel:

6. Emergency Obstetric Care at First Referral Unit (FRU):
   (a) What referral services at Community and Institutional levels are available:
   (b) Is there a blood storage centre at FRUs: Yes/No
   (c) Have the MBBS doctors got trained in life-saving anesthetic skills for emergency obstetric care: Yes/No
   (d) Have the MBBS doctors got trained in Emergency Obstetric Management skills: Yes/No
7. What safe abortion facilities do you provide:
   (a) Medical abortion under Medical Supervision
   (b) Provision of Quality Manual Vacuum Aspiration facility at the PHC
8. On ASHA (describe):
   (a) How many villages have ASHA
   (b) Do not have ASHA

Child Health:

9. What is the incidence/prevalence of Infant Mortality:
10. During the last year how many cases of these are reported:
    Acute Respiratory Infections (ARI):
    Diarrhoea: Measles: Malaria: Malnutrition:
11. How many neo-natal deaths are reported due to:
    Pre-maturity: Sepsis:
12. What measures were taken to promote breast feeding:
13. What measures were taken to promote complementary feeding and Micro-nutrients:
14. Have you followed any strategies of (a) strengthening the skills of health care workers:
15. Strengthening of health care infrastructure:
16. Involvement of Community
17. Describe the performance of ICDS
18. Anti malarial programmes
19. Home-based neo-natal care: Given/Not given
20. Do the CHWs/Nurses/ANMS got trained in resuscitate asphyxiated infants:

2. Immunization

21. Are the vaccinations to infants given for
    (a) Polio: Yes/No;
    (b) Diphtheria: Yes/No;
    (c) Pertussis: Yes/No;
    (d) Tetanus: Yes/No;
    (e) Measles: Yes/No;
    (f) Tuberculosis: Yes/No.
22. Are the pregnant women given during antenatal period: (i). Tetanus Toxoid Vaccination; (ii) Hepatitis B vaccine and (iii) injectable Vi Antigen Typhoid Vaccine
23. Did the children aged 12-23 months receive all primary vaccinations including measles by the age of one year:
24. In the light of Pulse Polio Campaigns, how many children received Polio Vaccine?
25. How many children aged 12-23 months received the vaccination for the following:
    BCG: Polio3: DPT3: Measles: All Vaccines:

3. Nutrition

26. How many children of 6-35 months are anaemic?
27. How many of married women in the age group 15-49 who are anaemic?
28. Is the Indian National Goitre Control Programme (NGCP) in operation?
29. How many cases of goitre (due to iodine deficiency) are reported?
30. Is iodized salt in supply?
31. How many Vitamin A Deficiency Disorders (VAD) such as corneal ulcers/softening of cornea (keratomalacia): Bitot spots are reported:

ICDS

32. What nutrition supplements are provided:
33. Describe the functioning of the Anganwadi centre in the delivery of primary health care interventions by the ANM such as immunization, distribution of Iron Folic Acid and Vitamin A supplements, distribution of oral contraceptive

pills and other contraceptives, growth monitoring and promotion, and health education and counselling to mothers:

34. Describe the Mid-Day Meal Programme:
35. Do the centres serve as immunization/antenatal care/ supplementary feed centres for 6 months to 2 years old children?
36. Are these services provided for children under:

	1 year	*1-3 years*	*3-6 years*
(i)Health check-ups	Yes/No	Yes/No	Yes/No
(ii) Immunization	Yes/No	Yes/No	Yes/No
(iii) Growth Promotion and Supplementary Feeding	Yes/No	Yes/No	Yes/No
(iv) Referral Services	Yes/No	Yes/No	Yes/No
(v) Early Childhood Care and Pre-school Education	Yes/No	Yes/No	Yes/No
(vi) Nutrition and health education	Yes/No	Yes/No	Yes/No

37. Describe the services provided for the following including health education:
    Adolescent Girls (11-18 years):
    Pregnant Women:
    Nursing Mothers:
    All Women (15-45 years):
38. Is there in operation National Nutritional Anaemia Prophylaxis Programme (NNAP) to prevent anaemia among pregnant women and children: Yes/No
39. Are iron and folic acid for 90 days distributed for pregnant women: Yes/No
40. Is there National Vitamin A Prophylaxis Programme for the Prevention of Blindness in operation: Yes/No
41. Describe the assistance given and the role of ASHA:

4. Prevention and Control of Locally Endemic Diseases

42. What is the prevalence/incidence of Tuberculosis among the tribals:

43. How many are covered under Directly Observed Treatment—Short Course (DOTS):—
HIV/AIDS:
44. Diarrhoeal Diseases Episodes per year:
45. Incidence of (a) Malaria: and (b) other Vector Borne Diseases such as— Filaria: Japanese Encephalitis: Dengue: Chickungunya: Leprosy:
Please list other endemic diseases in this area:
46. Is there indoor residual spraying with DDT:

5. Treatment of Common Illnesses and Injuries

47. Do the ANMs manning the sub-centre provided with prophylactic (Kit A) and essential drugs (Kit B) to manage commonly occurring illnesses and basic injuries in the community: Yes/No
48. Do the PHC/Sub-Centre staff got trained to diagnose and treat ARIs with oral cotrimoxazole:
49. How many deaths due to dehydration caused by acute diarrhoea reported:
50. Do the oral dehydration salt (ORS) solution administered: Yes/No
51. Do the tribal mothers being oriented to prepare and use the ORS solution at home when her child has diarrhoea: Yes/No
52. Are the ORS packets available with the ANM, AWW, and ASHA: Yes/No
53. Is there a supply of Zinc tablets as an adjunct to ORS: Yes/No
54. Has the community level link worker (ASHA) trained to deal with generic ailments at the village/hamlet level: Yes/No
55. Are the following provided with the drug kit to deliver first-contact health care:
(a) Kit A-IFA (large and small), Vitamin A solution,
(b) Cotrimoxazole tablets,
(c) ORS packets,
(d) disposable delivery kit;
(e) Kit B
(f) Methyl ergometrine Maleate tablets/Injection,

(g) Paracetamol tablets, Mebendazole tablets, and Dicyclomine tablets,
(h) Chloramphenicol eye ointment,
(i) Ointment Povidone Iodine,
(j) Cetrimide Powder,
(k) Cotton and bandages provided with a drug kit (including AYUSH drugs)

56. is the IMNCI followed as a standard operating procedures at the field level to manage neonatal and childhood morbidities: Yes/No
57. Do the health workers practice Syndromic-based diagnosis and management of reproductive tract infections/sexually transmitted infections (RTI/STI) at the field level: Yes/No
58. Do you have the supply of syndrome specific STI treatment kits to smoothen the treatment of RTI/STIs: Yes/No

6. Provision of Essential Drugs

59. Please list the essential drugs you need:
60. Are the drugs available on a regular basis:

(i). Yes/No
(ii). If No, Please give reasons:

61. Are the Sub-centers supplied with drug kits (Kit A and Kit B) every six months: Yes/No
62. How many drugs last beyond 6-8 weeks:
63. What strategies have been adapted for the safe and rational use of drugs:
64. Have the PHC staff got any in-service training: Yes/No
65. Have you got standard treatment guidelines: Yes/No

7. Water Supply and Sanitation

66. Do the para-medical staff address the question of sanitation in the villages: Yes/No
67. Do they impart any health education to the tribals: Yes/No
68. Are you aware of the list of essential drugs devised by Indian Public Health standard: Yes/No

8. Health Education

69. Do you know the treatment protocols for the following:

(a) TB: Yes/No
(b) Diarrhoea: Yes/No
(c) Leprosy: Yes/No
(d) Other immunization schedules: Yes/No

70. Do you engage in communication for behaviour changes to prevent HIV/AIDS and other life style diseases: Yes/No, If Yes, please describe:
71. List the IEC Interventions:
72. What in your opinion is the role of mass media:
73. Contextual needs if any specify
74. Is there any training health workers in interpersonal communication and campaigns
75. Do you monitor impact of IEC: Yes/No
76. Please describe the ASHA, ANM, AWW, VHSC Coordination:
77. Are there any health *melas* organized to spread health awareness among the tribals:
78. If so, please describe, when, where and how:
79. Do you think there are inherent drawbacks in the existing health programmes:
80. If so, please elaborate specifically:
81. How the out reach services can be improved, please suggest:
82. What in your opinion has to be immediately done to improve the performance of the PHC:
83. What could be the long term plans:
84. Please provide the staffing pattern, sanctioned, existing, including vacancies:

Bibliography

Ackernecht, Erwin H. (1942 b). "Primitive Medicine and Culture Pattern. *Bull., Hist. Med.*, xii 545-574.

Ackernecht, Erwin H. (1947). "Primitive Surgery." *Am. Anthrop.*, 49: 25-45l.

Alland, Alexander Jr. (1970). *Adaptation in Cultural Evolution: An Approach to Medical Anthropology*, Columbia University Press, New York.

Ali, Almas (1978). "Health and Genetic Problems of Kutia-Kondhs of Burlubaru Village, Phulbani District (Orissa)", Almas Ali in *Adivasi*, Vol. XVII, Nos. 1-4, April-July.

—— (1983). "Health Problems of Primitive Tribal Communities of Orissa", Dr. Almas Ali in *Adivasi*, Vol. XXIII, No. 2, July.

Behura, N.K. and K.K. Mohanty (2006). "Chapter 6: Ethno Medicines and Ethnic Healers in Sustainable Health Care Services: Case Studies from Tribal Societies of Orissa", pp. 100-143, in *Readings in Social Anthropology*, Dominant Publishers and Distributors, New Delhi, 2006.

Bulliyya, Gandham (2006). "Environment and Health Status of Primitive Paudi Bhuiyan Tribe in North Eastern Part of Orissa", pp. 336-368, in *Anthropology of Primitive Tribes in India*, P. Dash Sarma (ed.), Serials Publications, 2006.

Dunn, F.L. (1976). "Human Behavioural Factors in the Epidemiology and Control of Wuchereria and Brugia Infections", *Bull, Public Health Soc.*, Malay, 10: 34-44.

—— (1979)., "Behavioural Aspects of the Control of Parasitic Diseases", *Bull. of WHO*, 57: 499-512.

—— (1983). "Human Behaviour Factors in Mosquito Vector", Control". SE Asean J. Trop. Med Pub., *Health*, 14: 86-94.

Eliade (1951). "Referred in Royal Anthropological Institute, London", 1952, *Notes and Queries on Anthropology,* (ed.), G.P. Murdock, Routledge and Kegan Paul.

Elizabeth, K.M. and K.E. Rajpramukh (2000). "Potability of Water among the Tribals of Vizianagaram Sub-Plan Area, Andhra Pradesh: Microbiological and Physico-Chemical Analysis", *The Anthropologist*,12-3.

Foster, G.M. (1976). "Disease Etiologies in Non-western Medical Systems", *American Anthropologist*, 78: 773-782.

Gamango, A.K. (2007). "Ethnic Healers among the Dongria Kondh of Orissa", in *Adivasi*, Vol. 47, No. 1 and 2 June and Dec., pp. 139-149.

Goody, Jack (1962). *Death, Property and Ancestors: A Study of Mortuary Customs of the Lodagaa of West Africa*, Stanford, California, Stanford University Press.

Haribabu (2009). "Rural Health Care Delivery System and Health Infrastructure in Visakhapatnam District, Andhra Pradesh, India", in *Man and Life*, pp. 21-28.

Hemadri, K. (1994). *Sastravethalanu Akarshistunna Girijan Vaidyam* (Telugu), TCR and TI, Hyderabad.

Hemant Bag and Kapoor (2007). "Health Management among the Kondh: A Primitive Tribe of District Kalahandi, Orissa", in *Genes, Environment and Health—Anthropological Perspectives*, Serials Publications, New Delhi, 2007, pp. 37-48.

Hesser (1982). "Studies of Infectious Diseases in an Anthropological Context", *Med. Anthro.* 6: 1-10.

Hymavathi Devi J. (1996). Health, Illness and Treatment among the Kolams of Adilabad District, A.P, Unpublished M.A. Dissertation, University of Hyderabad.

Jhansi Rani (2009). The Bondo Women: Static Lives and Dynamic Roles. Unpublished Ph.D. Thesis submitted to Andhra University, Visakhapatnam.

Laxmi Narayan Dash, V. and T.S. Naidu (2007). *Food Habits and Nutritional Status of Eleven Tribes in the Four Southern States*, pp. 150-170.

Madhav Krishna, H. (1995). Culture and Illness among the Savara, unpublished M.Phil Thesis, University of Hyderabad, Hyderabad.

Mohanty G.N. and A.K. Mahapatra (2005). "The World of Saora Medicine: A Note on Belief System, Medicine and Medicineman", in *Adivasi*, Vol. 45, No. 1, June, pp. 1-11.

Mohanty, P.K. and P.K. Das (2007). "Nutritional Health Status of Selected Tribal Populations of Orissa: An Overview", pp. 52-61.

Mythili (1988). A Study on the Anthropometry of Tribals of Visakhapatnam Agency Area. Unpublished M.A. dissertation submitted to Andhra University.

Naidu, T.S. *et al.*, (2007). *Health Status of the Tribal Women and Children in India: A Case Study of Eleven Tribes of South India*. pp. 10-27.

Nanda, Kishore K. (1999). Culture and Illness among the Koya, Unpublished M.Phil Dissertation, University of Hyderabad.

Obeyesekere, Gananath (1969). "The Ritual Drama of the Sanni Demons: Collective Representations of Disease in Ceylon, Comparative Studies" in *Society and History* 11: 174-216.

Palanisamy, G. and T.S. Naidu (2007). *Family Planning Practices among the four primitive tribes of Nilgiri hills in Tamilnadu*, pp. 196-202.

Palgar (1962). "Health and Human Behaviour: Areas of Interest Common to the Social and Medical Science", *Current Anthropology*, 3: 154-205.

Quadeer, Imrana (1995). "Primary Health Care: A Paradise Lost", *IASSI Qrtly*, Vol. 14, Nos. 1 and 2, pp. 1-20.

Raj Pramukh, K.E. (1976). "A Note on the Shaman among the Jatapus", *Folklore* 17(2): 379-381.

Raj Pramukh, K.E. (1998). A Study on the Morbidities among the Tribals of Vizianagaram Sub-Plan Area, Andhra Pradesh, Unpublished Report—submitted to ITDA, Parvathipuram.

Raj Pramukh, K.E. (2005). "The Shaman in Asia Pacific Region, A Cross-cultural Study", *Man in India*, 85 (1 and 2) 25-40.

Rao, R.S. (2007) The evaluation of IFC services and Their Impact on the Tribal Communities of Visakhapatnam District Unpublished Report Submitted to TCR and TI, Hyderabad.

Rajan, S. *et al*. (2007). "Ethno-Medicine used by the Primitive Tribes of Nilgiris: An Emerging Trend in Phyto-ethnopharmacological Research", in *Tribal Health* (ed.) Naidu, T.S. pp. 259-270.

Roy, Aditya and B.V. Sharma (2005). "Ethnomedical Beliefs and Practices among the Saora, Chapter 32, pp. 454-464", in *Dimensions of Researches in Indian Anthropology* (ed.), Vijay S. Sahay, Pradeep K. Singh, Gautam K. Bora, Serials Publication, New Delhi.

Sankara Rao (2007). Sustainable Tribal Development: A Study in Gummalkshmipuram Mandal in Vizianagaram District of Andhra Pradesh. Unpublished Ph.D. Thesis, submitted to Andhra University, Visakhapatnam.

Sasicoumar Brumot, K. *et al.* (2007). Tobacco, Culture and Health Problems: A study among the Paniya Tribes of Nilgiri Hills, pp. 139-149 in *Tribal Health (ed.)* T.S. Naidu, Pondichery University.

Saurez, Maria (1974). "Etiology, Hunger and Folk Diseases in the Venezuelan andes", *Journal of anthropological Research*, 30: 41-54.

Snow, Loudell F. (1974). Folk Medical Beliefs and their Implications for Care of Patients *Annals of Internal Medicine* 81: 82-96.

Sujata Rao, K. (1998). "Health Care Services in Tribal Areas of Andhra Pradesh", *Economic and Political Weekly*, Feb. 28, 1998, pp. 481-486.

Veerraju, P. (1984). "A note on genetic disorders among the tribal groups of Andhra Pradesh" (pp. 142-152), in *Development Strategy, Primitive Tribal Groups* (ed.) by Ashokkumar Tigidi and K. Mohan Rao, TCRTI, Tribal Welfare Department, Government of A.P.

Venkateswarlu (1975). A Study of Dermatoglyphics on the Savara Males of Bhadragiri Agency in Srikakulam District of Andhra Pradesh. Unpublished M.A. Dissertation submitted to Andhra University.

Verma, R.C. (1990). *Indian Tribes Through Ages*. Ministry of Information and Broadcasting, Government of India, New Delhi.

Index